A Pocket Obstetrics

By the same authors

A pocket gynaecology
Tenth Edition 1983

A Pocket Obstetrics

Sir Stanley G. Clayton
MD MS (Lond.) FRCP FRCS FRCOG
Emeritus Professor of Obstetrics and
Gynaecology, King's College Hospital Medical
School, University of London. Honorary
Consulting Obstetric and Gynaecological
Surgeon, Queen Charlotte's Hospital and Chelsea
Hospital for Women, London.

John R. Newton
MD BS (Lond.) FRCOG
Lawson Tait Professor of Obstetrics and
Gynaecology, University of Birmingham.

TENTH EDITION

CHURCHILL LIVINGSTONE
EDINBURGH LONDON AND NEW YORK 1983

CHURCHILL LIVINGSTONE
Medical Division of Longman Group Limited

Distributed in the United States of America by
Churchill Livingstone Inc., 1560 Broadway, New
York, N.Y. 10036, and by associated companies,
branches and representatives throughout the world.

First Edition 1948   Sixth Edition 1967
Second Edition 1952   Seventh Edition 1972
Third Edition 1956   Eighth Edition 1976
Fourth Edition 1961   Ninth Edition 1979
Fifth Edition 1965   Tenth Edition 1983

ISBN 0 443 02008 6

British Library Cataloguing in Publication Data
Clayton, Stanley G.
  A pocket obstetrics. — 10th ed.
  1. Obstetrics
  I. Title   II. Newton, John R.
  618.2   RG524

Library of Congress Cataloging in Publication Data
Clayton, Stanley George, Sir.
  A pocket obstetrics.
  Bibliography: p.
  Includes index.
  1. Obstetrics — Handbooks, manuals, etc. I. Newton,
John Richard.   II. Title.   [DNLM: 1. Obstetrics — Hand-
books.   WQ 100 C625p]
RG531.C48   1983   618.2   83-2043

Printed in Singapore by
Huntsmen Offset Printing Pte Ltd.

Preface

This is an attempt to present the essential facts of obstetrics in a book that can literally be carried in the pocket. There has been a strict economy of words rather than omission of facts.

The present edition has been revised throughout to reflect the modern practice of obstetrics, with the more frequent use of the partogram, oxytocic infusions and fetal monitoring.

Facts are essential for obstetric practice, but understanding is also required, which cannot be derived from a book. It will only be gained by attendance on patients in the labour wards and clinics.

London 1983
S.G.C.
J.R.N.

Contents

1

Anatomy

Some points of normal anatomy which relate to obstetrics will be mentioned here. Other anatomical facts are given in later Chapters: bony pelvis (p. 24), fetal head (p. 26), placenta and cord (p. 8), fetal circulation (p. 10), changes in labour (p. 22).

The vagina

The vagina passes upwards and backwards, at a right angle to the axis of the uterus. The anterior wall is 7 cm long and is related to the urethra and the bladder. The posterior wall is 9 cm long and is related to the perineal body, the rectum and the recto-vaginal pouch (Fig. 1). The cervix projects into

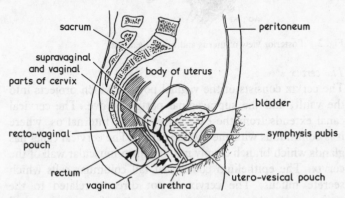

Fig. 1. Diagram of sagittal section of pelvis. (Arrows show direction of action of levator ani.)

the vaginal vault and divides it into four *fornices*. The shallow anterior fornix is related to the bladder, and the deep posterior fornix to the recto-vaginal pouch. Each lateral fornix is related to the base of the broad ligament, where the ureter and the uterine vessels lie. The vagina has a wall of smooth muscle and a lining of stratified epithelium without glands.

The uterus

The non-pregnant uterus is pear shaped and is 7.5 cm long (Fig. 2).It is divided into cervix (2.5 cm long) and body; the part of the body above the tubal orifices is the fundus. The fundus is normally directed forwards (*anteversion*).

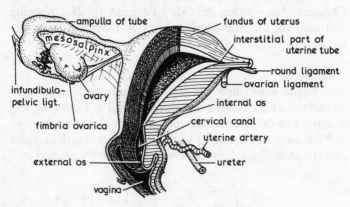

Fig. 2. Posterior view of uterus and broad ligament.

The cervix

The cervix consists of the vaginal portion which projects into the vault, and the supravaginal portion above. The cervical canal extends from the external os to the internal os, where it is continuous with the uterine cavity. The cervical canal has glands which branch deeply into the fibro-muscular wall of the cervix. The epithelium consists of tall columnar cells which secrete mucus. The cervix is not directly related to the peritoneum except on the posterior part of its supravaginal portion.

The body of the uterus

This is covered with peritoneum, except at a narrow area on either side, where the broad ligaments are attached. The wall is 1 cm thick, and consists of smooth muscle. The uterine cavity is triangular, with the apex inferiorly at the internal os, and with a tubal opening at each upper angle. The endometrium has simple tubular glands of columnar epithelium set in a vascular stroma. Unlike those of the cervix, the glands do not penetrate into the muscle coat. Cyclical menstrual changes occur in the endometrium.

Relations of the non-pregnant uterus

Anteriorly the peritoneum of the utero-vesical pouch covers the uterine body down to the level of the internal os, and below that the supravaginal cervix is related to the bladder. Posteriorly the uterine body is covered with peritoneum, which is continued downwards over the supravaginal cervix and vaginal vault. Laterally the uterus is related to the broad ligaments, and the ureter passes forwards 1 cm from the side of the cervix, with the uterine artery crossing above it.

The uterine (Fallopian) tubes

The two tubes extend outwards from the uterine cornua, and lie in the upper free edges of the broad ligaments. The part of the tube in the uterine wall is the interstitial portion, and is succeeded by the isthmus. The tube then widens out as the ampulla, and curves round the ovary before opening into the peritoneal cavity at the abdominal ostium. The tube has a complete peritoneal coat, except below where it is attached to the broad ligament, and a wall of smooth muscle. The ciliated epithelium is arranged in complex folds.

The ovaries

Each ovary is about 4 cm long, and is attached to the back of the broad ligament. The surface is covered with a single layer of cubical cells. The cortex contains the follicular elements scattered among the spindle-shaped stroma cells.

Ovarian (Graafian) follicles

The primitive follicle consists of a single large cell, the ovum, surrounded by a single ring of cells (Fig. 3). As the follicle ripens the cells around the ovum proliferate to become several layers deep, and are known as granulosa cells. As the granulosa cells increase in number a space containing fluid appears among them, so that the ovum is displaced to one side. Outside the granulosa cells is a layer of smaller theca-interna cells, and around these the stroma is condensed to form the theca-externa.

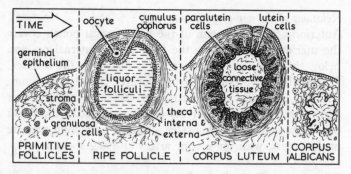

Fig. 3. Diagram of Graafian follicle and corpus luteum.

At birth the ovary contains thousands of follicles, but normally only one ripens fully in each menstrual cycle. This follicle approaches the surface of the ovary as it enlarges, and at ovulation the ovum is discharged into the peritoneal cavity. After ovulation the granulosa and theca-interna cells accumulate lipoid and become infolded into the cavity of the follicle, which is then called the *corpus luteum*.

The broad ligaments and pelvic cellular tissue

The broad ligaments are two transverse peritoneal folds which extend outwards from the lateral borders of the uterus to the pelvic wall on either side (Fig. 2). The uterine tube is in the upper free margin, and the ovary is attached to the back of the broad ligament. The base of the broad ligament widens out, so that the two peritoneal sheets of which it is composed are further apart, leaving a space containing loose cellular tissue.

All the spaces between the pelvic organs are filled with this loose cellular tissue, which is continuous with the extraperitoneal tissue of the anterior and posterior abdominal walls. The main mass of cellular tissue at the side of the uterus is known as *parametrium*.

Parts of the pelvic fascia are condensed to form ligaments which contain some unstriped muscle, and which support the uterus. The *cardinal ligament* (transverse pelvic ligament) extends from the side wall of the pelvis to the supravaginal cervix, and the *uterosacral ligament* passes backward from the cervix to the sacrum, lying to one side of the rectum.

The pelvic floor and perineal body

The lower third of the posterior wall of the vagina and the anal canal are separated by the *perineal body*. This is a pyramidal mass of muscle fibres, which come from the superficial perineal muscles, from the anterior part of the anal sphincter and from levator ani. The fibres cross the midline and interlace. *Levator ani muscle* arises from the back of the pubic bone, from the fascia on the side wall of the pelvis over obturator internus, and from the ischial spine. Its fibres pass backwards, downwards and inwards to be inserted into the perineal body, the anal canal, and the anococcygeal raphé. With its fellow of the opposite side the levator ani muscle forms a sling which draws the perineal body forwards and upwards. The urethra and vagina pass between the medial edges of the levator muscles. The function of the pelvic floor during labour is discussed on p. 29.

Blood supply of the pelvic organs

The ovaries, tubes and upper part of the uterus are supplied by the ovarian arteries, which are branches of the aorta and reach the fundus of the uterus in the upper margins of the broad ligaments.

The main supply to the uterus comes from the uterine arteries, which are branches of the hypogastric (internal iliac) arteries and pass medially in the bases of the broad ligaments.

The upper vagina is supplied by vaginal branches of the hypogastric arteries. The lower vagina and the pelvic floor are supplied by the pudendal arteries, which also arise from the hypogastric arteries, and run forward on the lateral wall of the ischio-rectal fossa, where inferior haemorrhoidal and perineal branches are given off.

Nerve supply of the pelvic organs

The uterus has a rich sympathetic supply from the pre-aortic and hypogastric plexuses, and also a parasympathetic supply from the sacral nerves. Normal uterine action will continue after division of the spinal cord, so the motor function of these nerves is uncertain.

Pain impulses caused by uterine contractions pass up the hypogastric nerves to reach the preaortic plexus and enter the cord as high as the 11th and 12th dorsal roots. Pain impulses from cervical dilatation also enter the cord by sacral roots. Injection of 20 ml of 1 per cent lignocaine into the extradural space, either by the lumbar route or through the sacral hiatus (caudal anaesthesia), will block these impulses.

Perineal pain impulses pass by the pudendal nerve, and slightly by the ilio-inguinal nerve. The pudendal nerve crosses the back (outer surface) of the ischial spine and then traverses the lateral wall of the ischio-rectal fossa. Pain pathways in the pudendal nerve can be blocked by injection of 10 ml of 1 per cent lignocaine near the ischial spine (*pudendal block*, p. 149).

The myometrium contains both α and β adrenergic receptors, as well as cholinergic receptors. The effect of adrenergic drugs on the uterus is variable, but strong stimulation of β receptors by β mimetic drugs such as isoxsuprine or Ritodrine will inhibit myometrial activity.

2

Normal pregnancy

Fertilization of the ovum and embedding

During coitus large numbers of motile spermatozoa are deposited in the upper vagina. A few enter the cervical mucus and ascend to the tube where conjugation of one of them with the oöcyte occurs. The fertilized ovum is carried down the tube by peristalsis and ciliary action. Ovulation occurs at about the 14th day of the cycle and the fertilized ovum reaches the uterine cavity about five days later.

In the first half of the menstrual cycle the endometrium grows thicker and more vascular under the influence of oestrogens from the ovarian follicle. In the second half of the cycle the corpus luteum secretes both oestrogens and progesterone, and these hormones cause secretory activity in the endometrial glands. The fertilized ovum reaches the uterus

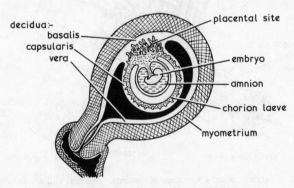

Fig. 4. Diagram to show embedding of embryo in decidua.

at this stage. The single cell has already divided actively and the outermost cells (*trophoblast*) are able to digest the superficial cells of the endometrium so that the ovum buries itself in the thickness of the endometrium, now called the *decidua* (Fig. 4). During pregnancy the corpus luteum persists for a time and its hormones assist in maintaining the decidua.

The placenta

The fetus soon develops its own heart and blood vessels and some of these vessels extend out of its body along the umbilical cord to the placenta. The placenta consists of numerous *chorionic villi*, each of which contains fetal blood vessels and is covered by trophoblast arranged in two layers — a deep layer of cuboidal cells (cytotrophoblast or Langhans' layer) and a superficial syncytium (syncytiotrophoblast).

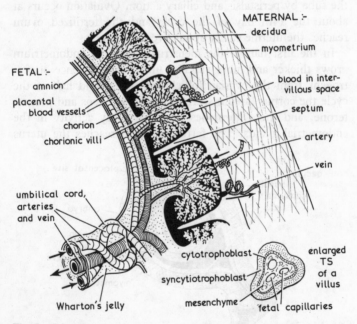

Fig. 5. Diagram to show structure of placenta. The real villi are far more complex and branched.

The majority of the villi branch freely in the intervillous space, but a few are attached to maternal decidua (Fig. 5). Maternal blood fills the spaces between the villi but does not mix with the fetal blood in the vessels in the villi, although if small injuries to the villi occur a few fetal red cells or fragments of villi may enter the maternal circulation.

In general the trophoblast and the endothelium of the villi form a semipermeable membrane, preventing the passage of substances of high molecular weight and particles such as bacteria, although some organisms (e.g. those of rubella, syphilis and toxoplasmosis) will invade the fetus. Blood gases and most substances of molecular weight less than 1000 pass freely, but the trophoblast has some selective activity. Some antibodies of very high molecular weight (e.g. rhesus antibodies) reach the fetus. Oestrogens, androgens, cortisone and thyroxine pass the placenta; insulin does not. Most drugs, antibiotics and anaesthetic agents will pass.

The placenta secretes chorionic gonadotrophin (p. 14), oestrogens (p. 64) and progesterone, and these hormones maintain the decidua and cause growth of the uterus and breasts. It also secretes corticotrophin and large amounts of lactogen (HPL*). The function of the latter is uncertain, but it has prolactin-like and growth-hormone-like activity. Little transfer to the fetus occurs.

The placenta is normally attached to the upper uterine segment. At term it weighs about 500 g and is about 20 cm in diameter. Sometimes the placenta has two lobes, and if one lobe is small and separate (*succenturiate lobe*) it may be retained when the rest of the placenta is delivered and cause postpartum haemorrhage.

The umbilical cord and membranes

The umbilical cord at term is usually about 50 cm long. It contains two arteries and one vein embedded in gelatinous mesodermal tissue (*Wharton's jelly*). When one artery is absent

* HPL = Human pracental lactogen.

the fetus sometimes shows other abnormalities. The cord is normally attached to the centre of the placenta, but sometimes joins the edge (*battledore insertion*). Rarely the umbilical vessels branch and run on the membranes before reaching the placenta (*velamentous insertion*), and if such a vessel lies below the presenting part (*vasa praevia*) it may be torn during labour.

The uterine cavity at term is lined by maternal decidua, and within that by *chorion*, a thick membrane (of which the placenta is a specialized part), and thin *amnion*. The amnion covers the placenta and umbilical cord, and is continuous with the fetal skin at the navel (Fig. 5). The amniotic cavity contains about 1200 ml of *liquor amnii*.

Fetal circulation

The two umbilical arteries carry blood to the placenta and are branches of the hypogastric (internal iliac) arteries. The umbilical vein returns oxygenated blood from the placenta to the portal vein, but much of this blood bypasses the liver through the *ductus venosus* to the inferior vena cava. The lungs are not functioning, and the pulmonary circulation is largely bypassed by two connections between the right and left sides of the circulation:

1. The *foramen ovale* between the two atria.
2. The *ductus arteriosus* between the pulmonary artery and aorta. When the cord is tied and respiration starts the pulmonary circulation opens up, and the foramen ovale and ductus arteriosus close.

Changes in maternal physiology

During pregnancy the uterus grows from a weight of about 60 g to 1000 g by proliferation and enlargement of the smooth muscle cells. The uterine blood vessels are enormously hypertrophied. Especially in the middle layer the muscle fibres are arranged in interlacing bundles which compress the large vascular sinuses when they contract, and so control bleeding after delivery.

The cervix and vagina become so vascular that they are softer and bluish in colour. The cervical glands proliferate and are so distended that the cervix appears to contain a plug of mucus.

The glandular structures of the breasts proliferate in response to oestrogens and progesterone.

During pregnancy the maternal basal metabolic rate increases by about 20 per cent, but in spite of that more weight is gained than is accounted for by the growth of the fetal tissues, the uterus and the breasts. The average gain is 11 kg. The rate of gain is greatest in late pregnancy, when it is about 0.5 kg per week. Part of the gain is water, and the blood volume increases, so that haemodilution occurs and the haemoglobin concentration falls (p. 76), but there is also a substantial gain in fat reserves.

The cardiac output rises by about 30 per cent, reaching this level by about the 28th week and so continuing to term. Peripheral vasodilatation occurs. There is often breathlessness, but the pulmonary vital capacity is not reduced.

The renal threshold for glucose often falls, so that sugar may be found in the urine although the blood sugar is normal (see p. 80). Dilatation of the renal pelves and ureters occurs, but there is no failure of renal function.

SYMPTOMS AND SIGNS OF PREGNANCY

Duration of pregnancy

The average duration of normal pregnancy is 282 days from the first day of the last menstrual period, i.e., 268 days from ovulation. The expected date of delivery can be estimated by adding seven days to the date of the LMP and subtracting three calendar months.

Symptoms and signs of normal pregnancy

Amenorrhoea

Pregnancy is the commonest cause of amenorrhoea during the child-bearing years. Slight bleeding may occur in early pregnancy, but such bleeding is unrelated to menstruation and should be regarded as abnormal, although often no harm results.

Morning sickness

Nausea or vomiting, usually only in the early morning, are common symptoms between the 6th and 14th weeks.

Breast changes

At six to eight weeks fullness and discomfort may be noted. In brunettes the areolae of the nipples become pigmented at about the 12th week; this change is permanent. Pigmentation may extend to skin beyond the areola (*secondary areola*) at about the 20th week; this will disappear after delivery. Areolar sebaceous glands become active (*Montgomery's tubercles*) and the nipples become more prominent. Clear secretion can be expressed at the 12th week and yellow colostrum near term. Once lactation has occurred secretion may persist, so that this sign is only useful in the diagnosis of a first pregnancy.

Changes in the skin

In some women stretching of the skin of the abdomen, and less often over the breasts, causes red lines (*striae gravidarum*). These persist but become white after delivery. There may be pigmentation in the midline of the abdomen (*linea nigra*) or on the face (*chloasma uterinum*): these signs will disappear after delivery.

Frequency of micturition

This may occur in early pregnancy because of pressure on the bladder by the uterus in the pelvis.

Changes in the vagina and cervix

These structures become so vascular that they appear blue and feel soft. There is an increase in vaginal secretion which may cause pruritus vulvae. The uterine isthmus softens before the lower cervix, so that on bimanual examination at about the

9th week the body and cervix of the uterus may feel as if they are separate structures (Hegar's sign).

Enlargement of the uterus

The body of the uterus becomes globular by about the 12th week, and it then rises up into the abdomen. Subsequently the fundus reaches the level of the umbilicus at the 24th week and the xiphoid cartilage at the 36th week. If the fetal head engages in the pelvic cavity the fundus may then descend a little ('lightening'). Painless uterine contractions occur and can be felt during pregnancy.

Signs due to the presence of the fetus

Fetal movements are usually felt by the mother ('quickening') at the 20th week, and may be felt later by the attendant. *Fetal heart sounds* can usually be heard with a fetal stethoscope at the 24th week. Occasionally a *uterine souffle* (a murmur due to blood flow in the uterine vessels) or a *funic souffle* (due to blood flow in umbilical vessels) may be heard. (Heart movements can also be recognized with ultrasound, p. 15).

Internal ballottement is a sign found on vaginal examination at about the 20th week, when the fetus may float upward in the liquor and then return to tap on the examining finger.

The various parts of the fetus can be felt and recognized by abdominal palpation in late pregnancy, and *external ballottement* may then be possible, when the fetal head can be displaced and then felt to return with a sharp tap. At this time fetal parts can also be distinguished on vaginal examination.

Other symptoms

Other symptoms which sometimes occur include vagaries of appetite, a dislike for smoking, constipation, tiredness, breathlessness towards term, and abdominal pruritus (see obstetric hepatosis, p. 85). Backache is common, but not always due to the pregnancy.

Laboratory tests

During pregnancy large amounts of chorionic gonadotrophin are secreted by the placenta and excreted in the maternal urine. A simple rapid pregnancy test can be performed on a glass slide in the clinic. Human gonadotrophin has antigenic properties, and on injection into animals antisera are produced. The steps of a typical test are:

1. Patient's urine is mixed with anti-HCG. If she is pregnant the urine contains HCG which neutralizes the anti-HCG.
2. The mixture is added to a suspension of particles coated with HCG.
3. If the patient is pregnant there is no reaction because the anti-HCG has been neutralized; if she is *not* pregnant the particles are agglutinated by the unfixed anti-HCG.

Such tests are only reliable 10 days after the first day of the last period, but pregnancy can be diagnosed immediately after a missed period by the more sensitive but more complex radio-immunoassay of β HCG in blood.

Radiological diagnosis

Fetal bones can be seen in a radiograph from the 16th week, but because of radiation hazards this method is not employed for the diagnosis of pregnancy.

Ultrasonic diagnosis

If sound waves of high frequency are directed through the body they are reflected at any interface between tissues of different physical properties. The returning waves permit echo sounding, so that the depth of interfaces can be measured. In the original A scan the degree of deflection of a dot of light on a screen indicated the strength of echo and this allowed measurement of distances between reflecting surfaces. In B scan the brightness of the dot varies according to the strength of echo, and by swinging the beam to and fro across the field a picture like that on a radar screen can be built up. In modern 'real time' machines a linear array or a rotating sector scan gives a continuous image resembling that of a television screen.

With ultrasound the gestation sac can be recognized within 5 weeks of conception, and very early diagnosis of multiple pregnancy is possible. The fetus can be made out from the 6th week, its crown-rump length measured from the 8th week, and the diameter of the fetal head from about the 12th week. The fetal head increases in size linearly until the 30th week, and records of early observations in a case with doubtful dates can be very useful later in pregnancy. After the 30th week the rate of growth is more variable, so that the scan cannot give a precise date, but it will indicate whether normal growth is continuing. Ultrasonic examination can also show fetal abnormalities such as anencephaly, spina bifida, cardiac lesions or polycystic kidneys.

The best and safest method of localizing the placenta is with ultrasound (See p. 69).

Another method of use of ultrasound allows recognition of fetal heart movements. When the waves strike a moving object such as the heart, or blood flowing in the placenta, the frequency of reflected waves is altered by the Doppler principle. With simple and easily portable machines fetal life can thus be demonstrated from about the 12th week.

ANTENATAL CARE

Good antenatal care reduces mortality and morbidity in the mother and the fetus. It includes:

1. *Detection and treatment of any intercurrent illness*, e.g. cardiac disease, diabetes, tuberculosis, pyelonephritis, syphilis or appendicitis. Some disorders begin before the pregnancy, others only arise or are discovered during it.
2. *Detection and treatment of complications of pregnancy*, e.g., antepartum haemorrhage, pre-eclampsia, anaemia or twins.

3. *Anticipation of complications of labour*, e.g., disproportion or malpresentations.
4. *Fetal considerations* include any foreseeable risk of fetal abnormality, e.g., prematurity, haemolytic disease, syphilis or placental insufficiency.
5. *Psychological preparation* for labour and instruction in the care of the baby.

A regular routine is essential. The mother's age, race, parity and social background are all important in obstetrics. At the first visit a *general medical history* is taken, including questions about cardiac disease, tuberculosis, diabetes, infection of the urinary tract and smoking habits. Any *previous obstetric history* is recorded, including for each pregnancy:

1. Any complications during pregnancy
2. Method of delivery and any complications, with the weight of the child, and
3. Any complications of the puerperium or infant feeding.

A woman who has had four previous pregnancies is often called a grand multipara. Such a patient tends to be older, and if her social conditions are poor she may have anaemia or poor nutrition. Because of the laxity of the uterus malpresentations may occur such as a transverse lie, uterine action may be weak during labour, and there is a risk of postpartum haemorrhage. After the age of 40 there is also an increased risk of Down's syndrome (p. 156).

The *history of the present pregnancy* is then taken, including the date of the last menstrual period, the regularity of previous cycles and (if applicable) the date of discontinuation of oral contraception.

General examination includes examination of the heart, lungs, breasts, legs and teeth. At the first visit a midstream specimen of urine is collected for bacterial culture (see p. 61). The urine is also examined for sugar and protein. If protein is found at any time a midstream specimen is taken to avoid vaginal contamination, and is examined for pus cells and organisms. The blood pressure is recorded, and blood is taken for haemoglobin estimation, grouping and serological test for syphilis. If the blood group is rhesus negative the blood is examined for antibodies. For Negro patients the haemoglobin type is determined by electrophoresis. The blood should also be tested for rubella antibodies (p. 82), and in many clinics the serum is routinely tested for alpha feto-protein (A-FP, see p. 156). A radiograph of the chest is taken if there is any suspicion of disease.

At *abdominal examination* the size of the uterus is noted, and in later pregnancy the position of the fetus and the fetal heart sounds. A *pelvic examination* is made to exclude any gross abnormality of the bony pelvis or pelvic organs. A cervical smear is taken for examination for cancer cells.

Subsequent visits should be monthly until the 30th week, fortnightly until the 36th week, and then weekly. At each visit the urine is examined for protein and sugar, the blood pressure is taken, and the legs and hands are examined for oedema. The patient is weighed regularly to detect excessive retention of fluid. In the later weeks abdominal palpation is regularly performed to find the fetal position (see below) and to exclude disproportion (see p. 101). It is wise to repeat the vaginal examination at the 36th week, as it is then easier to assess the size of pelvic cavity than in early pregnancy.

The haemoglobin concentration is estimated again at the 30th week and repeatedly if there is anaemia, and further antibody tests are done if the blood group is rhesus negative.

The full description of the fetal position includes the *lie* (longitudinal, oblique or transverse), *attitude* (flexed or extended, especially of the head), *presentation* (vertex, face, brow, breech or shoulder) and *position* (of the presenting part relative to the pelvis, e.g. left occipito-posterior position). The fetal heart sounds are usually heard through the back of the fetus, and lower in the maternal abdomen with a vertex than with a breech presentation. The presenting part is said to be *engaged* if its widest diameter has entered the pelvic brim.

The size of the fetus should, as far as possible, be assessed by careful palpation at each antenatal visit after the 28th week to detect any fetus that is 'small-for-dates' (see p. 166). If facilities are available the size of the fetus can be routinely determined by ultrasonic examination at booking and at the 28th week. If there is any doubt about fetal growth repeated ultrasonic measurement of the circumference of the fetal head and abdomen are made.

The mother may be asked to note the activity of the fetus, perhaps by counting the number of 'kicks' felt during one hour each day. If the count is low the case should be reviewed for any possible cause of placental insufficiency or fetal abnormality. A record of the fetal heart rate with an electronic ratemeter (see p. 33), using an external abdominal electrode, may be made over 30 minutes. The normal fetus has spells of activity during which the fetal heart rate shows variation, and the rate also responds to uterine contractions. Loss of these normal responses should cause anxiety.

Advice to the patient
It is convenient to give each patient a booklet as well as verbal directions.

Diet. An adequate intake of protein is needed (meat, fish, eggs, cheese). If fresh fruit and milk (1 pint daily) are added most vitamins and minerals will be adequately provided, but tablets containing ferrous fumarate (300 mg daily) and folic acid (0.3 mg daily) are given routinely.

Alcohol and *Smoking* should be strongly discouraged.

Teeth. Any carious teeth should be filled, and oral sepsis treated.

Bowels. Constipation is common and senna is effective.

Coitus. Coitus is unwise if there has been any bleeding, and in the last month.

Exercise. Exercise should be taken regularly, but over-fatigue avoided.

Breasts. Application of spirit or lanolin is useless; daily washing is all that is needed. If the nipples are flat, cups ('shells') may be worn under the brassière to press on the areolae.

Psychological preparation

Pregnant women may have many anxieties relating to health, labour, the unborn child and family relationships. Although 'old wives tales' are now less common, the press and television sometimes exaggerate problems and cause new anxieties. Ideal antenatal care would give time to deal with each individual patient's anxieties, but in the rush of hospital work this may be impossible and then antenatal mothercraft classes are invaluable, at which questions should be encouraged and carefully answered. The patient's general practitioner can play an important role in advising her.

In spite of loud claims, there is no scientific evidence that the course or safety of labour is altered by any form of antenatal exercises, although these may give confidence to those who believe in them.

If it is intended that the husband is to be with his wife during labour he should also be given preparatory instruction.

Selection of patients for hospital care

Although it is often claimed that it is as safe to have a baby at home as in hospital this is untrue, and reports which claim to show this are derived from groups of patients who are highly selected, both obstetrically and socially. The risk, especially to the fetus, is very high if an emergency arises at home during labour and the patient then has to be removed to hospital. If hospital beds are limited the following patients should have priority:

1. *Primigravidae*, who have an increased risk of pre-eclampsia, prolonged labour and operative delivery, and a relatively high perinatal mortality. The very young or the elderly primigravida needs special care.
2. *Grand multiparae*. After the fourth pregnancy the maternal risk exceeds that of a first pregnancy. The patients are older, and postpartum and antepartum haemorrhage, malpresentations and fetal abnormalities are more common.

3. Patients with a *history of obstetric abnormality* which may recur, such as hypertension, disproportion, and postpartum haemorrhage or the presence of a Caesarean scar.

4. Patients with *intercurrent medical disorders*, such as cardiac disease.

5. Patients who are found to have any obstetric abnormality in the current pregnancy, such as twins, antepartum haemorrhage or a malpresentation will require hospital treatment, but such abnormalities may not be evident at the time of booking.

6. If it is possible that a paediatric problem will arise it is essential that delivery should take place in a hospital with a fully equipped neonatal care unit. This includes patients with rhesus antibodies in their blood (p. 138).

General practitioners, provided that they have had basic practical obstetric experience, such as that gained in a six months resident hospital obstetric appointment, can play a useful part in obstetric care. Antenatal care may be shared with the hospital clinic, the doctor seeing the patient until the later weeks. Many patients can be delivered in G.P. obstetric units, provided that there is good liaison with, and close proximity to, specialist obstetric and paediatric services, and that patients with foreseeable abnormalities are not accepted.

DRUGS WHICH MAY AFFECT THE FETUS

The following drugs are occasionally harmful to the fetus and should only be used during pregnancy if there are good indications and no alternatives:

Long-acting *sulphonamides* interfere with the conjugation of bilirubin, *tetracyclines* may damage teeth, *streptomycin* may cause deafness, and *chloramphenicol* can cause postnatal collapse and hypothermia.

Ganglion-blocking drugs may cause neonatal ileus, *antithyroid drugs* fetal goitre, and *oral anticoagulants* placental haemorrhage. *Phenytoin* can interfere with folic acid metabolism.

Progestogens which have androgenic properties may cause masculinization of a female fetus, and *stilboestrol* vaginal carcinoma years later (in adolescence).

The following drugs can cause gross malformations and should *never* be given during pregnancy:

Thalidomide, cytotoxic and *alkylating drugs, radioisotopes.*

If given during late labour *morphine* or *pethidine* will depress the respiratory centre after delivery, but the effect can be counteracted with nalaxone (p. 160). *Diazepam* (Valium) will depress fetal cardiac and other medullary reflexes.

SMOKING AND ADDICTION DURING PREGNANCY

Heavy smoking during pregnancy, especially if there is also hypertension, is associated with fetal growth retardation and increased perinatal mortality.

Severe alcoholism may also be related to growth retardation. In cases of maternal heroin addiction the newborn infant shows withdrawal symptoms, with restlessness and failure to feed.

3

Normal labour

During pregnancy painless uterine contractions occur. When labour begins the contractions become stronger, more frequent and more regular. The pain is caused by ischaemia as each contraction arrests the myometrial blood flow. At the onset of labour the membranes over the internal os separate slightly and there is a little bleeding and discharge of mucus from the cervical canal (the '*show*'). Sometimes, especially if the presenting part does not fit well into the pelvic cavity, the membranes rupture early in labour.

The uterus has two functional divisions. The *lower segment* consists of the cervix and the lowest part of the body of the uterus. The rest is the *upper segment*, and this contracts more strongly than the lower segment so that the latter is gradually stretched and becomes thinner. The junction between the thick upper segment and the thin lower segment is *Bandl's retraction ring*.

The **cause of the onset of normal labour** is still uncertain. In sheep at term the fetal anterior pituitary secretes ACTH which causes the fetal adrenal cortex to liberate glucocorticoids which play a part in initiating labour. It is uncertain whether this is true for the human fetus, although pregnancy may be prolonged with anencephalic fetuses with abnormal adrenal cortices.

The evidence is against initiation of labour by oxytocin from the maternal or fetal posterior pituitary glands.

Placental progesterone may inhibit uterine activity during pregnancy, perhaps by blocking release of prostaglandin. At term high levels of oestradiol may stimulate release of prostaglandins from the myometrium and decidua.

The sensitivity of the myometrium to oxytocin or prostaglandins, or to stretching, increases as pregnancy approaches term. Over-stretching of the uterus (e.g., by twins) may cause premature labour, and rupture of the membranes will induce labour in late pregnancy.

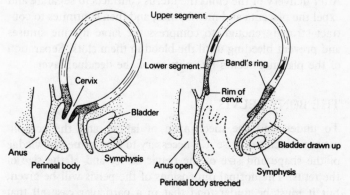

Fig. 6 Changes in uterus, vagina, perineum and adjacent structures during labour.

First stage of labour

This lasts until the cervix is fully dilated. During this stage the lower segment and cervix are drawn up over the contents of the uterus so that the cervix is first shortened ('taken up') and then dilated (see Fig. 6). As the supravaginal cervix is drawn up the bladder is carried up with it to become an abdominal organ. Between contractions the upper segment muscle fibres retain their tone, so that the fibres do not relax completely and any advance is held (*retraction*).

Second stage of labour

This lasts from full dilation of the cervix until delivery of the child. The membranes usually rupture during this stage and the presenting part descends into the vagina. The woman now uses her voluntary muscles to assist expulsion, holding her breath and pushing with each contraction. The presenting part descends on to the pelvic floor and the resistance of this directs the presenting part forwards under the subpubic arch to emerge through the vulval orifice. As the perineal body is stretched the anal orifice gapes.

Third stage of labour

After delivery of the child the uterus contracts to separate and expel the placenta and membranes, and then continues to contract strongly enough to compress the large uterine sinuses and prevent bleeding until the blood in them clots. Separation of the placenta occurs by splitting of the decidual layer.

THE BONY PELVIS

To understand the mechanism of labour and the complications which can arise it is necessary to have some knowledge of the shape and size of the pelvic cavity and of the size of the fetus. The normal dimensions of the pelvis will be given, but it must be understood that in a particular case all that matters is the relative size of the fetus to that of the pelvis. For obstetric purposes only the cavity of the pelvis, extending from the pelvic brim to the pelvic outlet, need be considered.

The pelvic brim

The plane of the brim is inclined at about 60° to the horizontal. It is bounded by a line running from the sacral promontory, along the sacral ala, across the sacro-iliac joint, and along the ilio-pectineal line and pubic crest to the back of the symphysis pubis (Fig. 7). The normal antero-posterior diameter (*true conjugate*) is 11 cm and the normal transverse diameter is 13 cm. In the living subject the true conjugate cannot be felt, but in cases of severe pelvic contraction the *diagonal conjugate* (from the lower margin of the symphysis to the promontory) may sometimes be determined by digital examination, and the true conjugate measures 1.3 cm less. In late pregnancy the best pelvimeter for the brim is the fetal head.

The pelvic outlet

The pelvic outlet is an imaginary plane passing through the lower end of the sacrum (*not* the coccyx) and the lower margin of the symphysis, and is inclined at about 20° to the horizontal. The ischial spines can be felt on the lateral pelvic wall just above this plane, and the ischial tuberosities lie well below it (Fig. 7). The subpubic angle is normally wider than 80°. The normal antero-posterior diameter of the outlet is 13 cm and the transverse diameter is 11 cm. The longest diameter of the

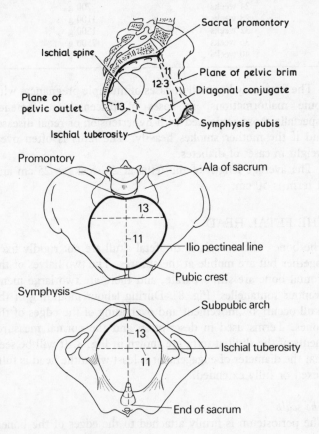

Fig. 7 Pelvic measurements. (cm.)

outlet is antero-posterior, whereas that of the brim is transverse. All the dimensions of the outlet can be estimated by vaginal examination.

FETAL WEIGHT AND MEASUREMENTS

Normal fetuses vary considerably in weight, but as a rough guide the following table is given:

24 weeks	700 g
28 weeks	1100 g
32 weeks	1500 g
36 weeks	2500 g
40 weeks	3500 g

The fetus may be small in cases of multiple pregnancy, with some malformations, in cases of placental insufficiency especially those associated with hypertension or renal disease, and if the mother smokes heavily. The fetus is often over-weight in cases of diabetes.

The average length of the fetus at 20 weeks is 25 cm and at term is 50 cm.

THE FETAL HEAD

The bones of the vault of the fetal skull are not rigidly fixed together but are mobile at the sutures. The two halves of the frontal bone are still separate, and there are two large membranous fontanelles (Fig. 8). During labour moulding of the skull occurs by movement and overriding of the edges of the bones. Terms used in description and the normal measurements of the skull at term are shown in Fig. 8. It will be seen that the diameter of engagement is least when the head is fully flexed or fully extended.

The scalp

The periosteum is firmly attached to the edges of the bones,

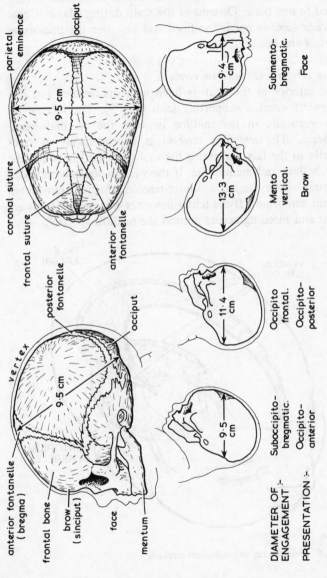

Fig. 8 Fetal head.

so that a subperiosteal haematoma (*Cephalhaematoma*) is confined to one bone. Oedema of the scalp during labour (*Caput succedaneum*) is not so confined and lies over the presenting part of the head.

Falx cerebri and tentorium cerebelli

The interior of the skull is lined with dura mater and this gives off internal supporting folds (Fig. 9). The *falx cerebri* lies vertically in the midline between the cerebral hemispheres. The *tentorium cerebelli* is approximately at right angles to the falx and forms the roof of a 'tent' in which the cerebellum and medulla lie. If the vault is strongly moulded during labour the falx is under tension which is transmitted to the tentorium. If the tentorium gives way nearby veins are torn and bleeding occurs around the medulla (p. 169).

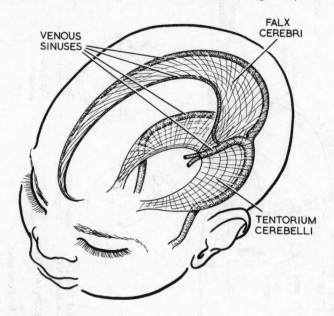

Fig. 9   Falx cerebri and tentorium cerebelli.

MECHANISM OF LABOUR

During its descent through the birth canal the fetus undergoes movements which are described as the mechanism of labour. At the onset of labour the head normally lies in the transverse or oblique diameter of the pelvis (Fig. 10). As the head descends it becomes more *flexed* so that the occiput becomes the lowest part of the head and impinges on the pelvic floor. The two levator ani muscles form a 'gutter' which slopes downwards and forwards in the midline. This gutter directs

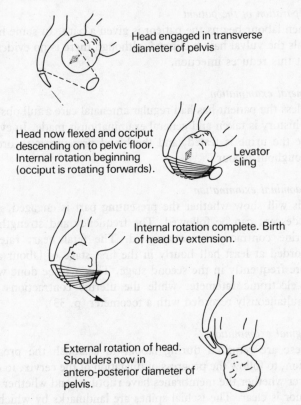

Head engaged in transverse diameter of pelvis

Head now flexed and occiput descending on to pelvic floor. Internal rotation beginning (occiput is rotating forwards).

Levator sling

Internal rotation complete. Birth of head by extension.

External rotation of head. Shoulders now in antero-posterior diameter of pelvis.

Fig. 10 Mechanism of normal labour.

the occiput forwards (*internal rotation*) so that it passes under the subpubic arch, and the head is born by *extension*. The shoulders remain in the antero-posterior diameter of the pelvis as they descend, so that the head is now at right angles to the shoulders. After delivery of the head it undergoes *external rotation*, to undo the twist of the neck. Delivery of the shoulders and trunk follows.

MANAGEMENT OF NORMAL LABOUR

Preparation of the patient

When labour begins the patient is given a bath. In some hospitals the vulval hair is clipped, although there is no evidence that this reduces infection.

General examination

Unless the patient has had regular antenatal care a full obstetric history is taken and general examination is made. In every case the urine is tested, and the blood pressure is recorded throughout labour.

Abdominal examination

This will show whether the presenting part is engaged, and its descent can be followed. The frequency and strength of uterine contractions are assessed. The fetal heart rate is recorded at least half hourly in the first stage of labour and more frequently in the second stage. This may be done with an electronic ratemeter while the uterine contractions are simultaneously recorded with a tocometer (p. 33).

Vaginal examinations

These are required during labour to establish the presentation, to follow the progress of dilatation of the cervix, to discover whether the membranes have ruptured and whether the liquor is clear. The ischial spines are landmarks by which to judge the degree of descent of the presenting part. Vaginal examination is preferable to rectal examination, which gives less accurate information. Vaginal examination is performed routinely at the onset of labour and when the membranes rupture — in the second instance to eliminate the rare possibility of prolapse of the cord. Examinations should be made at least 3 hourly, and more frequently when progress is in doubt.

Prevention of infection

Pathogenic bacteria may be introduced into the genital tract during labour and cause puerperal infection (see p. 125). Coliform bacteria are constantly present on the perineum, and staphylococci and streptococci may be widespread in a hospital, and these and other organisms may be carried on the skin or in the nose or throat of attendants. All who enter a labour ward should wear clean gowns and impervious masks, and these should be sterilized when worn for the conduct of the delivery, whether in hospital or elsewhere. Sterilized gloves are worn for any examination or operation, and in addition antiseptics should be freely used. Vulval pads must be sterilized and changed frequently.

In making a vaginal examination the genitalia are cleansed with swabs moistened with chlorhexidine solution (1:2000) passing each swab once from before backwards. The labia are separated and some chlorhexidine cream is placed around the vaginal orifice, into which the fingers are passed without touching neighbouring areas.

Progress of labour

Accurate records are essential for good obstetrics. The progress of cervical dilatation, the descent of the head, fetal heart rate, administration of drugs and other events in labour can be recorded on a time-sheet called a *partogram*, which is used to monitor the progress of labour. Figure 11 shows normal sigmoid curves for a primigravid and for a multigravid patient. There is first a 'latent phase', which is variable in duration but often lasts for about 8 hours from the onset of labour until the cervix is 4–5 cm dilated in a primigravida and 2–3 cm dilated in a multigravida. The 'active phase' follows

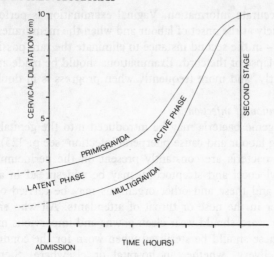

Fig. 11 Diagram of show normal progress of cervical dilation.

and lasts for about 3 hours during which the rate of cervical dilatation increases and should be not less than 1 cm per hour. There is sometimes a brief phase during which the rate of dilatation slows again before the second stage begins. In practical management the patient's partogram is compared with a normal curve; if progress is delayed her curve will be 'to the right' of normal.

Unassisted normal labour is always best and occurs in most cases, but if cervical dilatation does not occur at the normal rate the case needs special management. If progress is more than 2 hours delayed, and examination excludes serious disproportion or malpresentation, labour is 'augmented' by giving an intravenous infusion of 2 units of Syntocinon in 500 ml of normal glucose solution run at 40 drops per minute. The rate of the drip is regulated according to the uterine contractions, which must be carefully observed. Fetal death or uterine rupture can occur if the drip is not properly supervised, and the method is only suitable for fully staffed obstetric units, to which patients with delay in labour should be taken.

Automatic machines are available which regulate the infusion according to the rate of the contractions recorded by a toco-meter, but an ordinary drip can be used so long as the control is accurate. Fetal monitoring is desirable (see below).

Detection of fetal distress

The fetal heart rate is normally between 120 and 160 beats per minute. With fetal hypoxia the rate increases in a few cases, but a more serious sign which eventually occurs in every case is slowing, particularly after each uterine contrac-tion. Vagal impulses also cause the passage of meconium from the fetal bowel. Meconium is a dark green mixture of mucus, bile, intestinal ferments and epithelial debris. The passage of meconium is a less certain sign of fetal distress than slowing of the heart rate, but it always calls for careful assessment of the case.

In any high-risk case, and whenever there are clinical signs suggestive of fetal distress, special methods of fetal monitor-ing are used.

If the membranes have ruptured a small electrode can be attached to the fetal scalp to monitor the fetal heart rate from ECG signals. Alternatively the fetal heart movements can be monitored through the abdominal and uterine wall with an external electrode. Uterine contractions are recorded on the same trace by an external tocometer which is placed on the abdomen, or with an intra-amniotic catheter to measure intra-uterine pressure. 'Dips' in the heart rate may occur with uter-ine contractions. These decelerations are of little significance if the rate between contractions is normal, if they occur soon after the start of the contractions, and if the rate quickly returns to normal (Fig. 12). Decelerations which occur later after the start of the contractions and are prolonged are a warning of fetal danger, especially if there is also bradycardia between contractions. Such a trace would be an indication for taking a sample of fetal blood (see below). The heart rate nor-mally shows a beat-to-beat variation, and this is lost with hypoxia or deep sedation, so that the trace is flat.

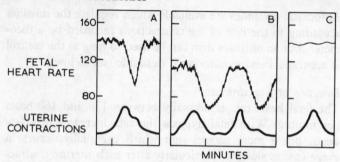

Fig. 12 Diagram to show traces obtained with fetal ratemeter.
A. Early deceleration occurring soon after uterine contraction.
B. Late and prolonged deceleration with basal bradycardia.
C. Flat trace with loss of beat-to-beat variation.

Apart from hypoxia, dips in the trace may also be caused by compression of the fetal head. Before any intervention such as Caesarean section the presence of hypoxia must be confirmed by examination of a sample of blood from the fetal scalp. To obtain this a tubular amnioscope is passed through the cervix and, after pricking the scalp, 0.3 ml of blood is collected with a fine heparinized tube. If there is hypoxia carbon dioxide accumulates and the fetal tissues begin anaerobic metabolism with conversion of glycogen to lactic acid, and the pH of the blood falls. The fetus is at risk if the pH lies below 7.20.

Normal first stage
During this stage the patient is more comfortable if she is up and about. When contractions become regular and if they cause distress an intramuscular injection of 200 mg of pethidine is given. Other drugs (e.g., promazine 50 mg) may be given in addition or as alternatives. In a long labour pethidine 100 mg may be repeated 2 hourly, but it should not be given if delivery is expected within that time. During labour reassurance is often required, and a patient should never be left alone in a closed room. Many women like to have their husbands with them.

Any patient in labour may require an anaesthetic unexpectedly and nothing should be given by mouth which, if vomited and aspirated, could obstruct the air passages. Only fluids or sieved food should be given. In a long labour the urine is tested for ketone bodies, and if these are present an intravenous infusion of glucose is given.

In the first stage progress is assessed by the dilatation of the cervix, which should be thin and well applied to the presenting part. If the membranes remain intact when labour is established they are ruptured with a pair of toothed forceps.

Epidural analgesia may be started in this stage, and continued until delivery. Alternatively inhalation analgesia may be used when the first stage is well established (see below).

Normal second stage

During this stage the patient is kept in bed. It is important that the general atmosphere of the labour room should be calm and quiet; le Boyer has recently re-emphasized the importance of this. The dorsal position may be the best for 'pushing'. In a few patients this position causes 'supine hypotension' because the uterus compresses the inferior vena cava and impedes venous return; if there is fetal distress the patient should be placed on her side. If the patient desires it, pain may be relieved by an inhalation of nitrous oxide and oxygen, or trilene with air is given with each contraction. Special machines have been devised which only deliver mixtures of analgesic gases when the patient holds the mask over her face and breathes deeply. Cylinders which contain a mixture of equal parts of nitrous oxide and oxygen ('Entonox') are available. In addition a pudendal nerve block (see p. 149) or infiltration of the perineum with lignocaine (1 per cent) may be used, unless an epidural injection has already been given.

In this stage progress is judged by descent of the presenting part, and eventually by bulging of the perineum.

For delivery the dorsal position is now commonly used in hospital, but elsewhere, with little assistance and no adequate method of supporting the legs, the left lateral position is better. Sterilized towels are arranged and antiseptic cream is freely applied to the vulva. If the bladder is full a catheter is passed.

There are a few patients who demand to be delivered in 'natural' positions, standing, crouching, or on their hands and knees. While their right of choice cannot be denied, it must be explained to them that there is danger to the child if the fetal heart rate is not regularly observed, and that care of the perineum is hardly possible in such positions.

Delivery of the head

To prevent tearing of the perineum the attendant must maintain flexion of the head with his hand until it is crowned (i.e. the parietal eminences are free), and must control the rate of delivery. Once the head is crowned it is delivered slowly between pains when the uterus is relaxed. If the perineum threatens to tear or if there is any delay an episiotomy is performed. The incision starts in the midline and then passes backwards and laterally to avoid the anal sphincter.

Delivery of the shoulders

The perineum is often damaged by the shoulders and vigilance should not be relaxed at this moment. If a loop of cord is around the neck this is either slipped over the head or clamped and cut.

The head is first drawn towards the sacrum to make sure

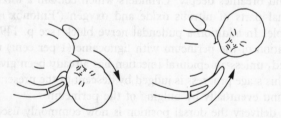

Fig. 13 Delivery of shoulders.

that the anterior shoulder has passed under the subpubic arch (Fig. 13). The head is then drawn towards the symphysis and the posterior shoulder usually sweeps over the perineum. If it does not do so traction is made with a finger in the posterior axilla.

An intravenous injection of ergometrine or an intramuscular injection of Syntometrine is given as soon as the delivery of the shoulders is safely under way (see Third Stage below).

Immediate care of the child

As soon as possible the pharynx is cleared with a mucus aspirator, even before delivery of the shoulders if someone is free to do this. The child is kept at the same level as the placenta in the uterus until the cord ceases to pulsate. The cord is then clamped or tied in two places and then cut at least 5 cm from the umbilicus. For the action to be taken if respiration is not immediately established see p. 161. Unless resuscitation is required the baby should at once be given to the mother to see and hold, possibly even before the cord is cut. le Boyer has stressed the importance of immediate close 'skin to skin' contact between the mother and her baby, which promotes emotional bonding. A normal baby should always be kept closely beside its mother.

Third Stage

If no assistance is given in the third stage, the uterus usually remains quiescent for some minutes. It then contracts to separate the placenta completely and to expel it from the upper segment into the dilated lower segment and vagina. With normal retraction of the upper segment the uterine vessels in its wall are compressed and there is only slight bleeding. The patient may be able to expel the placenta from the vagina by contraction of her abdominal muscles.

Signs of separation

When the placenta has separated and the uterus is contracting the fundus feels hard and globular, is mobile from side to side, and rises in the abdomen. The cord lengthens, and there may be a gush of blood, normally of less than 100 ml.

Active management

It is now the general practice to assist the third stage actively, except in cases of hypertension (see below), because this reduces the average blood loss and, more importantly, the number of cases of severe bleeding. Directly the anterior shoulder of the fetus is safely past the subpubic arch, the mother is given either ergometrine 0.5 mg intravenously, or Syntometrine (a mixture of Syntocinon 5 units and ergometrine 0.5 mg) intramuscularly. Intravenous ergometrine acts almost at once; intramuscular ergometrine takes about 4 minutes to act and for that reason the Syntocinon, which acts more quickly, is included in Syntometrine.

With either method the uterus contracts strongly and the placenta separates almost at once and is delivered by the *Brandt-Andrews method*. The patient must be in the dorsal position. The attendant stands on her right side and places his left hand just above the symphysis pubis. Upward pressure is maintained with this hand to displace the uterus from the pelvis. This avoids the risk of inversion while steady downward and backward traction on the cord is made with the other hand. There should be no delay in delivery of the placenta after giving ergometrine; otherwise there is a slight risk of the placenta being retained by strong contraction of the lower segment.

The Brandt-Andrews manoeuvre is to be distinguished from "expression" of the placenta by squeezing the fundus violently. This may cause shock, is ineffective, and will cause bleeding if the placenta is only partly separated.

In patients with hypertension ergometrine is not used unless abnormal bleeding occurs, because there is some risk of increasing the blood pressure and causing postpartum eclampsia. In such cases placental separation is awaited before delivering it by Brandt-Andrews method.

In all cases the placenta and membranes are examined after delivery and the placental weight should be recorded. If any part of the placenta is missing the uterus must be explored. Incomplete membranes are of less consequence. The number of cord vessels should be noted; when one artery is absent there are often fetal abnormalities.

Before leaving the patient the attendant must see that all bleeding has stopped and that the uterus is well contracted.

4

Normal puerperium

The puerperium is the period after delivery during which the genital organs return to their ordinary state. It lasts about six weeks.

Involution of the uterus
The large vessels in the uterine wall are occluded with blood clot and a new system of smaller vessels develops by organization of the clot. Rapid autolysis of the muscle cells occurs. After delivery the fundus is about 12 cm above the symphysis, but the uterus becomes impalpable in the abdomen by the 10th day. The cervix also becomes closed in this time, and the pelvic floor soon regains its tone.

Lochia
Decidual remnants, except for the basal layer from which regeneration of the endometrium occurs, are discharged in the lochia. At first the discharge chiefly consists of red blood cells, but later it becomes paler and contains more leucocytes. Red lochia continue for at least 10 days. Excessive bleeding occurs when placental tissue is retained. The lochia become offensive with some bacterial infections.

Breasts
During pregnancy the ducts and acini of the breasts proliferate. The ducts contain *colostrum*, a yellow fluid containing many fat globules and with a high protein content. Secretion of milk does not occur until after delivery when the hormone

prolactin is released from the anterior pituitary gland. On the fourth day after delivery acute engorgement of the breasts may occur when secretion begins. Stimulation of the nipple by the infant causes reflex secretion of oxytocin by the posterior pituitary gland, and this not only causes uterine contractions ('*after-pain*') but also contraction of myoepithelial cells around the acini and the consequent outflow of milk, described by veterinarians as the 'let down' reflex.

General metabolic changes

All the changes of pregnancy such as increased metabolic rate, increased cardiac output, fluid retention and changes in the renal tract are quickly reversed, except that most women have gained weight. Some of this is lost during lactation.

MANAGEMENT OF THE NORMAL PUERPERIUM

Prevention of infection

The temperature and pulse rate are recorded as these will give early warning of infection of the genital or urinary tract.

Aseptic technique is continued in the puerperium. Sterilized vulval pads are worn and frequently changed. Vaginal douching is harmful, and vulval 'bathedowns' are of no value in preventing infection. As soon as patients are up they may use a bidet or bath themselves. Nevertheless precautions against cross-infection must be strict, and any infected patient is isolated and her toilet facilities kept separate.

Sleep and rest

Undue excitement or insomnia should be treated with hypnotics. In the early puerperium a transient attack of depression, with weeping, is common; it only calls for sympathetic reassurance. More persistent depression or aversion to the baby must be taken more seriously (see p. 134).

Patients with no complications are allowed up within a few hours, but they should have at least 10 days rest from housework. Early ambulation reduces the risk of venous thrombosis without any evident increase in the incidence of prolapse.

Too many visitors should not be allowed. In hospitals children are sometimes excluded because of the risk of infection, but this rule is founded on theory rather than any adverse experience.

In hospital physiotherapists can teach exercises for the abdominal and pelvic floor muscles, which patients may continue at home.

Hospital stay
Provided that the patient's doctor and the community midwife are available to surpervise them at home, fit mothers and babies can be discharged after 48 hours or much earlier, although many normal patients stay for 5 to 6 days which has the advantage that lactation can be established before discharge.

Diet
The same diet as that recommended during pregnancy is appropriate, but abundant fluid is required during lactation.

Bowels
For constipation senna or cascara may be used, or an enema given. Aperients in excess may affect the baby through the milk.

Retention of urine
This sometimes occurs after difficult delivery, especially if there is pain from perineal stitches, and catheterization is then required.

Breast feeding
See p. 164.

POSTNATAL EXAMINATION

The patient should be examined before discharge from hospital and at six weeks after delivery. The latter examination is usually made by the general practitioner. The purpose is to detect any pelvic abnormality that has resulted from the pregnancy or labour, and to follow up such complications as cardiac disease, hypertension, urinary tract infection or anaemia. Advice on infant feeding may be required, and every patient should be asked if she needs family planning advice, which can then be arranged. See 'Pocket Gynaecology', Chapter 8.

Apart from the investigation of specific complaints, abdominal and vaginal examinations are made, and a speculum is passed. Abnormalities found come into the field of gynaecology but the following are common:

Retroversion of the uterus
If this was known to be present before the pregnancy, or if there are no symptoms, it needs no treatment. Only in exceptional cases with pelvic discomfort is a Hodge pessary inserted to hold the uterus forwards until involution is complete.

Cervical erosions
These should not be treated at the sixth week as most of them resolve. The patient is seen again at the 12th week, and only if the erosion persists and causes discharge is cervical cauterization or cryosurgery advised.

Prolapse and stress incontinence
Pelvic floor exercises may effect some improvement, but most cases eventually require surgical treatment.

Backache
Backache is common but seldom due to pelvic disorders. It is more often due to postural defects which are made worse by fatigue.

5

Abnormal pregnancy

ABORTION

Abortion is defined as the expulsion of the conceptus before the 28th week of pregnancy. The majority of cases occur during the first 12 weeks, when the entire product of conception is separated by haemorrhage and expelled by painful uterine contractions. In later abortion the mechanism resembles that of labour; after rupture of the membranes, the fetus is expelled by uterine contractions, followed by the placenta.

Causes

1. *Fetal abnormality* is the commonest cause of early abortion. Chromosomal abnormalities are found in more than a third of these cases.
2. *Uterine abnormalities*, including congenital malformations, fibromyomata, retroversion (only in cases of incarceration), deep cervical tears or amputation of the cervix.
3. *Maternal illness*, including acute fever, chronic nephritis, diabetes. Syphilis sometimes causes late abortion.
4. *Drugs*. Lead, ergot, quinine, cytotoxic drugs. Purges and oxytocics (except prostaglandins) usually have little effect.
5. *Trauma* has little effect on normal pregnancy, unless the uterine cavity is entered by some instrument.
6. *Hormone deficiency*. An uncertain cause (see p. 46).

Types of abortion

Threatened abortion
Slight bleeding occurs, but soon ceases, and the pregnancy

continues. Ultrasonic examination will show an intact gestation sac, and later in pregnancy the fetus can be shown to be alive by detection of its heart movements by ultrasound. The patient is kept at rest in bed until fresh bleeding has ceased.

Inevitable abortion

An abortion is judged to be inevitable when severe bleeding occurs, or slighter loss continues for more than about three weeks; when there is much pain; when the cervix is dilated; or when any part of the uterine contents is expelled. If there is doubt whether abortion is threatened or inevitable ultrasonic examination is helpful. Estimations of levels of chorionic gonadotrophin or of progesterone give variable results which may be inconclusive.

In a *complete abortion* everything is expelled and bleeding soon stops. In *incomplete abortion* bleeding continues and there is greater risk of infection. In a few cases the embryo dies, but is retained for some time — *missed abortion* (see below). Treatment of inevitable abortion: Give ergometrine (0.5 mg intramuscularly). Examine carefully anything that is passed, to avoid doubt whether the abortion is complete or incomplete. Surgical evacuation is essential for severe or continued loss, and wise if the abortion is still incomplete after 12 hours. The cervix is gently dilated and the contents of the uterus are evacuated with a suction cannula or with ring forceps under scrupulous asepsis. Blood transfusion may be necessary.

Sepsis may follow or accompany any abortion, especially criminal abortion, in which there may also be injuries such as perforation of the uterus. There is pyrexia and foul discharge, and septicaemia, peritonitis, cellulitis or salpingitis may occur. Ampicillin and metronidazole are given while awaiting the bacteriological report on a high vaginal swab. If there is urgent bleeding exploration of the uterus with ovum forceps to remove retained chorionic tissue cannot be delayed, but if the bleeding is slight this can be postponed until chemotherapy has had effect. Also see bacteraemic shock (p. 123).

Missed abortion (carneous mole)

Slow bleeding occurs into the chorio-decidual space, raising hillocks of clot that project under the amnion. The embryo is killed but not expelled at once. There is a history of a few missed periods, but the uterus does not continue to enlarge. Slight bleeding may continue. Pregnancy tests may be weakly positive as long as any chorionic villi survive. The risk of sepsis is small and spontaneous delivery can be awaited. There is a very remote risk of hypofibrinogenaemia (p. 117). An intravenous infusion of oxytocin or prostaglandins may be tried, and surgical evacuation is only considered after some weeks.

Repeated abortion

May be due to:

1. Maternal chronic illness; chronic nephritis, syphilis.
2. Uterine malformation or cervical incompetence.
3. Fetal abnormalities.

Apart from these cases the term *habitual abortion* is applied to cases of repeated abortion with no evident cause. Progesterone deficiency has been assumed to cause poor development of the decidua. Good results have been claimed after the intramuscular injection of hydroxyprogesterone caproate (Primolut Depot) 125 mg twice weekly, or of chorionic gonadotrophin (HCG) 10 000 units three times a week. However, there is no convincing evidence that this is effective. With some other progestogens there is a slight risk of causing virilization of a female fetus.

Since at least 10 per cent of pregnancies end in abortion for a variety of reasons, out of 1000 women who become pregnant twice, 10 women would be expected to have two successive miscarriages by mere chance, and would probably succeed in a third pregnancy even without treatment. Care must therefore be exercised in studying claims that a particular treatment is effective. Rest in bed, for several weeks if necessary, may be as effective as endocrine treatment.

Obstetrical injury or injudicious dilatation may cause *incom-*

petence of the cervix. Abortion from this cause usually occurs in the middle trimester of pregnancy, with almost painless dilatation of the cervix, and rupture of the bulging membranes. A torn cervix may be repaired; in other cases a purse-string suture of fascia or silk may be placed in the cervix during early pregnancy.

Legal termination of pregnancy See 'Pocket Gynaecology' Ch. 9.

Prevention of haemolytic disease
All rhesus negative patients are given anti-D globulin 100 μg intramuscularly within 48 hours after abortion.

VESICULAR (HYDATIDIFORM) MOLE

In this condition abnormal proliferation of the trophoblast covering the chorionic villi occurs, and cystic degeneration occurs in the central stroma of the villi. Fetal blood vessels are scanty, and no embryo is found. The uterus is full of grape-like vesicles. About 10 per cent of vesicular moles become malignant; the trophoblast gives rise to chorion-carcinoma (see below). Both moles and chorion-carcinomata secrete large amounts of chorionic gonadotrophin, and this causes the formation of multiple theca-lutein cysts in the ovaries. This disorder is common in Asia and West Africa.

The cells of most moles have the chromosomal complement 46xx, but studies of the banding of the chromosomes and of cell antigens suggest that the chromosomal material is all derived from sperm. Some error in fertilization or cell division has clearly occurred, but its nature is still uncertain.

Clinical features
After a variable period of amenorrhoea (often about 16 weeks) there may be bleeding, sometimes with a watery discharge and occasionally with the escape of vesicles. The uterus is often (but not always) larger than expected, without any of the usual signs of the presence of a fetus. The patient may feel ill, with vomiting, hypertension or proteinuria. Enlarged

ovaries may be felt. The laboratory tests for pregnancy are usually positive, even when the urine is diluted 1:100. Spontaneous abortion of the mole may occur.

The diagnosis can be confirmed by ultrasonic examination.

Management

The mole should not be allowed to remain. If it is not expelled with an intravenous infusion of oxytocin or prostaglandins an anaesthetic is given, and the mole is evacuated with a suction catheter after dilatation of the cervix. Abdominal hysterotomy is sometimes recommended, but is no safer. If the patient is over 40 or desires no more children hysterectomy (with the mole *in situ*) reduces the risk of subsequent chorion-carcinoma.

Regular estimations of the blood levels of chorionic gonadotrophins must be made by radioimmunoassay afterwards, first at six weeks and then three monthly for at least three years. If the test remains or becomes positive, or if there is any irregular bleeding, chorion-carcinoma is strongly suspected, provided that another pregnancy has not occurred.

CHORION-CARCINOMA

This highly malignant growth spreads by the blood stream to brain, lungs and liver, and locally to the pelvic structures and the vault of the vagina, where a vascular nodule may be seen. Many cases respond to treatment with the folic acid antagonist methotrexate. This is given orally in 7-day courses of 20 mg daily. As the drug depresses the bone marrow regular white cell counts are required during treatment. In addition actinomycin D or other chemotherapy is often given.

ECTOPIC PREGNANCY

The ovum is normally fertilized in the uterine tube. Embedding sometimes occurs in the tube instead of the uterus, and in extremely rare instances in the ovary.

Aetiology

Mild pelvic infection (occasionally tuberculous) may damage the tube without causing complete obstruction, and so impede the onward passage of the ovum. In the last 10 years there has been an increase in the incidence of pelvic infection, including that caused by *Chlamydia*, and there have been more cases of ectopic pregnancy.

There is also a higher incidence of ectopic pregnancy in women who have previously used an intrauterine contraceptive device, presumably because of mild pelvic infection.

However, in many cases of ectopic pregnancy no cause is evident.

Pathology

Tubal pregnancy is commonest in the ampulla, but may occur anywhere in the tube. The zygote burrows through the tubal mucosa into the muscle wall, where its enlargement splits the wall into two laminae. The tube cannot hypertrophy to accommodate the growing embryo and eventually the gestation sac gives way with the following alternative results:

External tubal rupture

The sac ruptures outwards.

1. *Intraperitoneal rupture*. Usually rupture occurs into the peritoneal cavity with free bleeding. Haemorrhage may be torrential, or slower when blood collects beside the tube (paratubal haematocele) or runs down to collect in the recto-vaginal pouch (pelvic haematocele).
2. *Intraligamentous rupture*. Less commonly rupture occurs into the space between the layers of the broad ligament (intraligamentous haematoma).

In both intraperitoneal and intraligamentous rupture the embryo usually dies, but rarely it retains sufficient attachment to survive as a secondary *abdominal or intraligamentous pregnancy*.

Internal tubal rupture

The sac ruptures into the tubal lumen. The embryo, together with blood clot, may be retained in the tube (*tubal mole*) or expelled through the abdominal ostium by muscular contractions (*tubal abortion*). In either case blood escapes from the ostium and may collect nearby (peritubal haematocele) or run down to the recto-vaginal pouch (pelvic haematocele).

In response to the pregnancy hormones the empty uterus enlarges and decidual formation occurs. When the embryo dies the decidua breaks down and uterine bleeding occurs. Laboratory tests for pregnancy are positive for a time.

In very rare cases in which the fetus survives, the placenta becomes attached to bowel or other adjacent structures, which become matted to the gestation sac. Fetal abnormalities are common. At term uterine contractions ('false labour') are followed by fetal death. A retained dead fetus may become calcified (*lithopaedion*), or infection may occur with formation of an abscess containing fetal bones.

Clinical features

These chiefly depend upon the amount and rate of intra-peritioneal bleeding. There is:

1. Usually amenorrhoea — one or two periods missed, seldom more.
2. Always pain.
3. After a few hours, uterine bleeding.

Cases with severe intraperitoneal flooding

Although this picture is classical it is less common than that of slower bleeding (below). There is severe abdominal pain. The patient collapses and may faint or vomit. In severe cases air hunger or even death occurs. On examination there is pallor, with a rapid pulse and low blood pressure. The abdomen is tender and distended, and sometimes rigid. Since the tube has ruptured completely and the blood is still fluid, no swelling is felt on vaginal examination.

Cases with slower bleeding

This is the commonest type of case. One or two periods are missed, then recurrent or persisting attacks of pain occur, with vaginal bleeding. Passage of a decidual cast is rare. The patient is pale and the pulse rate is increased. The temperature is often slightly raised. There is lower abdominal tenderness, and on vaginal examination a very tender swelling is felt in one postero-lateral fornix (tubal mole or a haematocele).

Pelvic haematocele

A few cases are first seen with a large haematocele after several days of abdominal pain. Pallor and slight fever are usual. A large pelvic mass of uneven consistency is found displacing the uterus forwards and the bowel loops upwards. Retention of urine may occur. A pelvic abscess sometimes follows.

Secondary abdominal pregnancy

This is very rare and may be undiagnosed for a time. There is usually a history of abdominal pain in early pregnancy. The fetus is felt unusually easily, and its position is often abnormal on radiological examination. The empty uterus may be felt separately from the gestation sac.

Diagnosis

Cases with severe bleeding are usually obvious. Cases with slower bleeding may be confused with:

1. Uterine abortion. In these cases there is no tubal swelling; bleeding precedes pain and is more profuse.
2. Torsion of an ovarian cyst. There is no evidence of pregnancy and the well-defined tumour is felt.
3. Appendicitis. There is an 'alimentary' history, with fever and right-sided pain.
4. Salpingitis. There is a history of the cause, with vaginal discharge, high fever, bilateral pain and swellings.

If there is doubt, ultrasonic examination may be helpful, but usually examination under anaesthesia and laparoscopy is essential. If a mass is felt beside the uterus the abdomen should be opened.

Treatment

In cases with rapid intraperitoneal bleeding operation is urgent. A ruptured tube is so damaged that it has to be removed. As bleeding often continues or recurs, much delay for resuscitation is unwise; transfuse and operate simultaneously.

In cases with slower bleeding operation is less urgent. An untreated tubal mole or haematocele may absorb, but without operation diagnosis is often uncertain and there is a risk of further bleeding or infection. In some of these cases the damaged tube may be conserved after removal of a mole.

If a pelvic haematocele becomes infected it may be drained vaginally, otherwise the abdominal route is better.

For secondary abdominal pregnancy laparotomy is performed to remove the fetus. If the placenta is much attached to structures such as bowel it may be left to absorb. Delay to allow the fetus to mature is unjustifiably hazardous, especially as the fetus may be malformed.

VOMITING DURING PREGNANCY

Vomiting at any stage of pregnancy may be due to any intercurrent illness, which a full clinical examination should discover. Pyelonephritis is a common cause, but rarer causes such as intestinal obstruction or a cerebral tumour occasionally occur.

Nausea or occasional vomiting occurs in about a third of normal pregnancies during the first trimester. Although called morning sickness it is not always confined to the early morning. The patient's health is not disturbed and vomiting stops spontaneously at about the 14th week.

Morning sickness may be related to the high levels of chorionic gonadotrophin which are found at this stage of pregnancy. Vomiting is more severe with twins or vesicular mole, when high levels of gonadotrophins are found.

In a few cases the vomiting is more frequent and it may persist beyond the 14th week, and disturb the patient's health (hyperemesis gravidarum). This exaggeration of a 'normal' symptom usually has a psychological cause. It may symbolize a wish to reject the pregnancy, or may be a demonstration to evoke sympathy. The vomiting nearly always stops when the patient is removed from her home and admitted to hospital without any other treatment. Ptyalism (excessive salivation) is of a similar nature.

Although excessive vomiting starts as a psychological illness the patient can eventually become physically ill, with dehydration, loss of salt, and ketosis due to starvation. The urine contains acetone bodies. In exceedingly rare instances there is polyneuritis and encephalopathy due to deficiency of vitamin B_1. Hepatic necrosis has been described, but in most cases the liver only shows fatty infiltration.

Management

Simple cases respond to reassurance, sometimes with the help of antihistamine tablets, such as meclozine 25 mg thrice daily, or promethazine theoclate 25 mg thrice daily. There is no good evidence that these drugs harm the fetus.

Severe cases are admitted to hospital. The few patients who do not improve immediately are given intravenous glucose and saline infusions as required to maintain a urinary output of about 1 litre with a salt content of at least 3 g daily. Oral feeding is resumed as soon as possible. Aneurin hydrochloride 10 mg is sometimes injected intramuscularly. In recent years, with adequate control of water and salt balance, termination of pregnancy is hardly ever necessary on purely medical grounds. Social and psychological problems may call for help.

HYPERTENSION AND PROTEINURIA

Hypertension or proteinuria may be due to pre-existing disease which is discovered or intensified during pregnancy, such as essential hypertension (p. 59), chronic nephritis (p. 60) or pyelonephritis (p. 60). Other much rarer causes include aortic coarctation, polycystic kidneys, phaeochromocytoma,and lupus erythematosus. Yet it is common for hypertension and proteinuria to appear in late pregnancy in women who neither then nor subsequently show evidence of any of these diseases, and (for want of a better term) these cases are described as pre-eclampsia, because a few of them progress to eclamptic convulsions. The term 'toxaemia' was formerly used when eclampsia was thought to be caused by a toxin. The words 'pregnancy induced hypertension' are non-committal.

Pre-eclampsia and eclampsia (Pregnancy induced hypertension)

Aetiology and pathology
It is convenient to discuss these after describing the clinical features. See p. 58.

Clinical features
Signs precede symptoms and usually occur after the 28th week. The disease is more common in teenage primigravidae, in women over 35 and in twin pregnancies, and may occur with vesicular moles. The signs resolve quickly after delivery, and sometimes before delivery if the fetus dies. The chief signs are:

Hypertension. Any rise of blood pressure of 20 mm Hg systolic or 10 mm diastolic above the pressure recorded in early pregnancy is suspicious, e.g. a pressure of 130/80 mm in a patient with an initial pressure of 110/70 mm. In severe cases the pressure may exceed 200/140 mm.

Fluid retention. Slight oedema of the ankles may occur in normal pregnancy, but severe oedema of the ankles, or oedema of the hands or face are signs of abnormal fluid retention. A weight gain of more than 1 kg in a week is also suspicious.

Proteinuria occurs in more severe cases, and may be heavy. Blood or casts are not found in the urine, and the blood urea concentration and renal function tests are usually normal except in cases of eclampsia. A midstream specimen is always obtained and examined to exclude of pyelonephritis.

Symptoms only occur in cases in imminent danger of eclampsia. *Headache and vomiting* may occur when the diastolic pressure is over 100 mm. *Visual disturbances* are caused by retinal oedema, and *epigastric pain* may be caused by hepatic subcapsular haemorrhages. Jaundice may result from hepatic necrosis.

The fetus. Particularly in cases with proteinuria or long-continued hypertension the fetus may be underweight, and it may die in the uterus. Gross placental lesions are rarely found, but it is assumed that there is spasm of maternal blood vessels supplying the placenta. There may also be fibrin deposition in the intervillous space. Neonatal death may also occur from prematurity.

Eclampsia. The progress of pre-eclampsia is extremely variable; most cases are mild but a few progress very rapidly to eclampsia when repeated fits occur, with deep coma between the convulsions. Eclampsia may also occur in the first 24 hours after delivery, but such *postpartum eclampsia* is usually mild. With repeated fits death may occur from cerebral haemorrhage, heart failure and pulmonary oedema, liver failure, or anuria due to renal necrosis (p. 134).

Management of pre-eclampsia

No effective prevention is known, but early detection by antenatal care will prevent dangerous progression. Patients with a persistent or increasing rise of blood pressure, especially if there is oedema, and all those with proteinuria are admitted to hospital for observation. There is no satisfactory treatment. Although termination of the pregnancy is often required to halt the disease, the fetus fortunately is usually viable except in a few cases of early onset.

Rest in bed is believed to increase the uterine blood flow and also to reduce the blood pressure.

Diet. A normal diet with adequate protein is given.

Fluid and salt. There is no good evidence that salt restriction alters the underlying disease process, but in cases with severe oedema the salt intake may be reduced and oral frusemide 80 mg daily may be given. A normal fluid intake is allowed.

Hypotensive and sedative drugs. Many drugs will lower the blood pressure but it yet to be shown that they improve the fetal prognosis. Drugs such as propranolol and methyl dopa have a limited place for exceptional cases when severe and progressive hypertension occurs before the fetus is large enough to survive delivery. For acute hypertension hydrallazine 30 mg intravenously may be used. In severe cases diazepam (Valium) 10 mg every 6 hours may be injected as a sedative and anticonvulsant, but this drug has a severe depressant effect on the fetus. The doses of these drugs are adjusted according to their effects.

Except in very mild cases the state of the fetus must be monitored:

1. By repeated ultrasonic measurement.
2. With placental function tests such as urinary oestriol estimations.
3. By observation of the fetal movements and variation in the fetal heart rate (p. 18).

Termination of the pregnancy is indicated when:

1. The hypertension or proteinuria, although not particularly severe, increases in spite of rest.
2. The blood pressure is at such a high level that eclampsia is feared, especially if heavy sedation for 24 hours has had no effect.
3. In all cases at or near term.
4. If the fetus is not growing, especially if there has been an intrauterine death in a previous pregnancy. A low urinary oestriol excretion is an additional sign of placental insufficiency.

In nearly all multigravidae, and in most primigravidae after the 35th week, labour is induced by low rupture of the membranes. If there is not rapid progress a Syntocinon drip may be used. Although there is a possible risk of increasing the blood pressure the drip is often preferable to Caesarean section. During labour and for a few hours afterwards the blood pressure must be watched, as a further rise may occur and should be controlled with hypotensive and sedative drugs. For primigravidae at 34 weeks or less, and for severe cases at later stages in which labour does not follow induction, Caesarean section is considered.

Treatment of eclampsia

All cases are removed to hospital. It is best if a strong sedative (see below) is given first, and the doctor must travel with the patient to treat any respiratory difficulty which may arise.

Sedatives. Many drugs have been recommended to control the fits. Two alternatives are:

1. Diazepam (Valium) 10 mg is given intravenously and subsequent doses adjusted according to effect. The patient is kept deeply sedated until the fits are controlled.
2. A slow intravenous infusion of chlorpromazine 35 mg, phenergan 50 mg and pethidine 100 mg in 50 ml of 50 per cent dextrose solution; this may be followed by intramuscular injections of half of these doses every three hours.

Hypotensive drugs have been mentioned above.

Diuretics. Intravenous frusemide 60 mg can be given if there is gross oedema.

Nursing care. Any disturbance may precipitate another fit, so the patient is kept in a quiet room. Some manipulations are unavoidable. The patient must be turned from time to time to prevent pulmonary collapse. An indwelling catheter gives accurate knowledge of her urinary output. Blood pressure, pulse rate and fluid balance must be recorded frequently.

During a fit restraint may be needed, and a mouth prop may prevent the tongue being bitten. If the patient is unconscious nothing is given by mouth, and if there is vomiting gastric aspiration is required. A suction machine, laryngo-scope and oxygen must be available. Antibiotics are given if she is long unconscious to prevent pulmonary infection.

Delivery. Some patients are already in labour; otherwise, after control of the fits, labour is induced by rupture of the membranes. Caesarean section is recommended if delivery is likely to be difficult or delayed for any reason.

Prognosis

The immediate maternal risk is slight unless eclampsia occurs, but then the mortality may be 5 per cent except in postpar-tum cases, in which it is lower. The fetal mortality in pre-eclampsia is about 3 per cent, but rises to over 30 per cent in eclampsia.

If a patient has pre-eclampsia in one pregnancy she has a 50 per cent chance of it in a subsequent pregnancy, but if she has it in two pregnancies the subsequent incidence rises to over 75 per cent. Such patients with 'recurrent toxaemia' probably have essential hypertension (see below) which has been unmasked by the pregnancy. Pre-eclampsia or eclampsia are not followed by chronic nephritis, and it is not believed that they make essential hypertension worse. The patient who subsequently has hypertension would probably have had it in any case.

Pathology

The morbid anatomy is unknown except in fatal cases of eclampsia; the pathology of pre-eclampsia is uncertain. In eclampsia the liver shows haemorrhagic necrosis of the peripheral (portal) parts of the lobules. In the kidney swelling of the glomerular endothelium and degeneration of the tub-ules may be found; renal necrosis is rare. Cerebral haemor-rhage may cause death. Pulmonary congestion and signs of heart failure are usual. Widespread intravascular micro-coagulation may occur.

Aetiology

The cause of pre-eclampsia and eclampsia is unknown. The underlying features of both are vasoconstriction and fluid retention. It would take the whole of this book even to list the theories of causation which have been put forward. No theory has so far led to successful prevention. The most fashionable theories at present are:

1. That relative uterine ischaemia in late pregnancy causes the release of vasoconstrictor substances from the uterus and placenta which act either directly or by reflex effect on the kidney.
2. That the vascular system gradually becomes sensitized by the hormonal changes of pregnancy.
3. That widespread intravascular coagulation causes renal, hepatic, cerebral and placental lesions. While this may be true in eclampsia the evidence is unconvincing in pre-eclampsia.
4. Abnormal maternal immune response to the fetus is possible, but as yet unproven.

Essential hypertension in pregnancy

Cases of hypertension which are discovered in early pregnancy, and for which no underlying cause is found, are placed in this category. There is often a family history of hypertension. From experience the obstetrician regards any blood pressure over 130/80 mm with suspicion, although a physician (who is thinking only of cardiac, renal and cerebral disease) would disregard it.

It is found that patients with an initial blood pressure of more than 130/80 mm have a 60 per cent probability of a rise of pressure in late pregnancy, when proteinuria may appear. This is described as 'pre-eclampsia superimposed on essential hypertension'. The course of events and the management are the same as in pre-eclampsia, except that the trouble is likely to recur in every successive pregnancy, and that there is likely to be progressive hypertension in later life. In rare cases the hypertension progresses rapidly, but in most cases the immediate maternal prognosis is good.

Some of these patients will already be taking hypotensive drugs before pregnancy; these are usually continued. Otherwise the management is the same as for pre-eclampsia.

Chronic nephritis

Nephritis is a rare complication of pregnancy; its course is probably unaffected by pregnancy. The diagnosis rests on the history and the discovery of proteinuria, oedema or hypertension in early pregnancy.

Some patients give a past history of acute nephritis. If they only have proteinuria the maternal and fetal prognosis is good, but if the disease has progressed to severe hypertension the maternal prognosis is already bad, and intrauterine fetal death often occurs.

Other cases are of insidious onset. If there is severe oedema and proteinuria the maternal and fetal prognosis is bad, but patients with only slight proteinuria and good renal function tests usually do well during pregnancy.

The management is similar to that of pre-eclampsia; early termination of pregnancy is only required for severe and progressive cases.

Lupus erythematosus

The maternal and fetal prognosis is bad in pregnancy, even if steroids are administered.

Acute pyelonephritis

Aetiology and pathology

The infection is nearly always due to *E. coli* which enters the bladder from the urethra and multiplies there. If the vesico-ureteric sphincter is ineffective infected urine reaches the renal pelvis, causing acute infection which always involves the substance of the kidney. The infection may precede pregnancy, often dating from childhood and being followed by recurrent attacks of 'cystitis', but in other cases it first occurs during pregnancy. Routine testing of midstream specimens in the antenatal clinic shows that about 5 per cent of pregnant women have more than 10^5 *E. coli* per ml in the urine in early pregnancy, and about half of these pateints with *asymptomatic bacteriuria* will develop acute pyelonephritis later in pregnancy. During pregnancy the ureters and renal pelves become dilated and atonic, partly as a progesterone effect and partly from pressure from the uterus, and urinary stasis occurs.

After acute infection small foci of infection may persist in the kidney and cause bacilluria and also lead to chronic pyelonephritis, with patchy fibrosis and ultimate renal failure or hypertension.

Clinical features

Symptoms most commonly appear after the 20th week. In severe cases there is fever (sometimes high, with rigors), pain in the loin (most frequently on the right) and vomiting. There may be no frequency or pain on micturition, but a midstream specimen contains many pus cells and organisms, and occasionally blood. Anaemia is common. Fetal death may occur in severe cases, and in chronic cases the fetus may be underweight.

Differential diagnosis

Appendicitis. In pyelonephritis pain is usually in the loin and bilateral, but with ureteric inflammation there may be iliac pain. In a case severe enough to mimic appendicitis the urine will contain many pus cells.

Pre-eclampsia. In any case of proteinuria midstream urine should be examined for pus cells and bacteria. In pyelonephritis there is no hypertension unless there is long-standing renal damage.

Anaemia. Renal infection should be excluded in any case of anaemia that does not respond to treatment.

Treatment

The patient is put to bed and given a light diet with extra fluid. Ampicillin 500 mg 6-hourly and metronidazole 1 g twice daily, are given. Most cases respond within about five days, but otherwise or if unusual organisms are found, and if sensitivity tests dictate, then other antibiotics are used. Repeated examination of the urine is essential to ensure that the urine is made sterile and remains so. In persistent cases an intravenous pyelogram is performed about 12 weeks after delivery to exclude other renal abnormalities.

Prophylaxis. In antenatal clinics every patient should be examined for bacilluria early in pregnancy. If it is found treatment is given with sulphonamides or the appropriate antibiotic. Repeated courses may be required.

HYDRAMNIOS (More correctly Polyhydramnios)

The mechanism controlling the volume of liquor amnii is not understood. The fluid is constantly being secreted and reabsorbed; part of it is swallowed by the fetus and excreted through the placenta. Fetal urine only makes a small contribution. Excessive liquor (polyhydramnios) is found:

1. In one sac with uniovular twins.
2. With fetal abnormalities. In cases of anencephaly and oesophageal atresia this may be because swallowing does not occur, but hydramnios occurs with other defects.
3. With placental angiomata; this very rare event shows that fluid can come from fetal vessels.
4. With maternal diabetes, when fetus and placenta are both large.
5. With hydrops fetalis (p. 139).

   Often no cause is found.

Clinical features

   Acute hydramnios is rare, and usually associated with uniovular twins. It occurs at about 20 weeks and causes painful uterine distension. Abortion usually occurs.

Chronic hydramnios is far more common, and is found after the 30th week. There is discomfort and breathlessness, but not pain. The uterus is larger than expected from the duration of gestation. It is difficult to feel or hear the fetus and (in contrast to twin pregnancy) the uterus feels full of fluid rather than of solid fetuses. Radiological and ultrasonic examination is essential to exclude twins or fetal abnormalities, although not all abnormalities can thus be detected. If amniocentesis is performed the fluid should be examined for alpha-fetoprotein (see p. 156). The urine is tested for sugar.

There is an increased incidence of pre-eclampsia. The membranes may rupture or labour may start prematurely. Malpresentations or cord prolapse may occur. The duration of labour is usually normal, but postpartum haemorrhage may be caused by poor uterine retraction. The total fetal mortality is high, from prematurity, abnormalities, diabetes and mal-presentations. If the fetus has any difficulty in swallowing after birth an oesophageal tube should be passed to exclude atresia.

Treatment
Rest in bed may relieve discomfort. If there are severe symptoms before the 36th week abdominal paracentesis may be tried. Fluid is taken off slowly through a fine needle. After the 36th week the membranes may be ruptured and an oxytocic drip set up, especially if the fetus is known to be abnormal. There is a slight risk of placental separation if a lot of liquor suddenly escapes.

Oligohydramnios
The volume of liquor is relatively less in late pregnancy. Oligohydramnios is also associated with the fetal abnormality of renal agenesis.

PATHOLOGY OF THE PLACENTA

Near or after term the trophoblast covering the chorionic villi often shows degenerative changes and as a result maternal blood around these villi may clot or deposit fibrin. Calcification is common near the decidual plate. The placental reserve is so great that these degenerative changes seldom affect the fetus. Cysts and tumours (angiomata) are rare.

In diabetes and haemolytic disease the placenta is large. The placenta may be infected by syphilis.

Placental insufficiency may occur in pre-eclampsia, hypertension, renal disease, postmaturity, diabetes, if the mother smokes heavily and in other cases without explanation. Sometimes intrauterine fetal death occurs in successive pregnancies.

Placental function tests

Placental insufficiency during pregnancy may be recognized by:

1. *Failure of fetal growth*. This may be observed clinically and by repeated ultrasonic examination.
2. *Measurement of placental hormones*. Oestriol assay is at present the best test. The formation of oestriol is a complex process. Dehydroepiandrosterone is produced by the fetal adrenal, hydrolysed by the fetal liver, and converted to oestriol in the placenta. The oestriol passes into the maternal blood and is finally excreted by the maternal kidney.

Maternal plasma oestrogen may be estimated as an index of oestriol production, or the oestriol output can be measured in the urine, in which it rises progressively to about 25 mg daily at term.

If the fetus is anencephalic with defective suprarenal glands little oestriol will appear; with twins an increased amount may be excreted. With placental failure and associated defective fetal metabolism the excretion may be low or fall. The range of normal variation is wide and repeated observations are essential. Any placental function test may be wrongly interpreted if the fetal maturity is uncertain.

An alternative test is to measure the blood level of HPL (lactogen) which is formed by the placenta.

ANTEPARTUM HAEMORRHAGE

Antepartum haemorrhage is defined as bleeding from the placental site after the 28th week of pregnancy and before the birth of the child. It may come from:

1. A normally situated placenta — Abruptio placentae (accidental haemorrhage).
2. A placenta situated wholly or partly on the lower uterine segment — *Placenta praevia*.

Vaginal bleeding in late pregnancy may also come from an erosion, polyp or carcinoma of the cervix. Such *incidental bleeding* will cause diagnostic difficulty but is not usually included in the conventional definition.

ABRUPTIO PLACENTAE (Accidental haemorrhage)

Aetiology
Pre-eclampsia or hypertension are found in association with 30 per cent of the cases, but it is uncertain whether these cause the haemorrhage; in some cases proteinuria and hypertension follow rather than precede the bleeding.

Abruptio placentae occurs most frequently in patients with a poor social and nutritional background, and folic acid deficiency has been found in some of these cases. Claims that prophylactic administration of folic acid will prevent the disease are unconfirmed.

In a small number of cases placental separation is due to trauma such as external version, but in most cases there has been no injury, and the word 'accidental' is only used in contrast to the 'unavoidable' haemorrhage of placenta praevia.

Pathology

When retroplacental bleeding occurs there may be a localized haematoma, or extensive separation of the placenta which will kill the fetus. A large collection of blood may track down between the membranes and the uterine wall to escape through the cervix (*revealed bleeding*), or it may be retained within the uterus (*concealed bleeding*), and mixed types occur.

In cases of severe concealed haemorrhage blood not only collects behind the placenta but infiltrates into the wall of the uterus, disrupting the muscles fibres and even reaching the peritoneal surface (Couvelaire uterus). In some of these cases disorders of blood coagulation occur (p. 117). Some cases are followed by anuria, probably due to arterial spasm from a utero-renal reflex, but which may end with renal necrosis (p. 134).

Concealed haemorrhage

Clinical features

Severe cases are fortunately uncommon, as the patient is severely shocked and may die. She is pale and complains of severe and continuous abdominal pain. The pulse rate may be rapid, but is not always so, even when the patient is obviously very ill. The uterus is tender to the touch, distended and may feel hard. It is difficult to feel the fetus, but in late pregnancy the head is often engaged. The fetus is almost invariably dead and the heart sounds are not heard.

With a small retroplacental haemorrhage the patient complains of pain and there is localized tenderness, but there is little or no shock and the fetal heart sounds may be heard.

Treatment

In a severe case morphine is injected at once and blood transfusion started. The pulse rate and arterial blood pressure should not be the only indications of the amount of blood needed; measurement of the central venous pressure is the best guide. In cases that respond to treatment labour often starts spontaneously, but if it does not then the membranes are ruptured, and if contractions do not follow a Syntocinon drip is started.

If the patient is still very ill and labour is not in progress a difficult decision has to be made. Caesarean section obviously carries a grave risk, yet if the patient is left she may die undelivered.

In any case postpartum haemorrhage may follow. This may respond to the usual treatment, but if the blood does not clot the temperature discussed on p. 117 is required. Hysterectomy is a desperate measure which is seldom justified.

In slight cases of concealed bleeding the diagnosis is often uncertain. Admission to hospital for observation is essential, and if there is any evidence of fetal distress Caesarean section is performed.

Revealed haemorrhage

Clinical features

In severe cases there is uterine tenderness and the fetal heart sounds are absent; with the bleeding the diagnosis is obvious. In slighter cases in which the only sign is bleeding the differential diagnosis from placenta praevia is often difficult. If the head is engaged placenta praevia of serious degree is excluded. The position of the placenta can be determined by ultrasonic examination. *All cases, however slight, should be admitted to hospital for observation, without pelvic examination.*

Treatment

If there has only been slight loss and the fetal heart sounds are normal no immediate treatment is necessary until the differential diagnosis has been resolved. If placenta praevia can be excluded and no further loss occurs the patient is only kept at rest for a few days.

If the loss is heavy and there is much pain the fetus is

usually dead. Blood transfusion is begun. Unless labour is in progress the membranes are ruptured. If a placenta praevia cannot be excluded this is done in the operating theatre under anaesthesia with all preparations made for Caesarean section. If contractions do not follow rupture of the membranes an oxytocic drip is set up.

Caesarean section is only recommended for the unusual case in which bleeding is heavy, labour is not in progress and the fetus is alive.

PLACENTA PRAEVIA

Aetiology and pathology

The reason for low implantation is unknown. It occurs in about 1 in 200 pregnancies, and the incidence increases slightly with advancing age and parity. A placenta praevia is often thinner and more adherent than a normal placenta.

Degrees

Four degrees have been described:

Type I: (Lateral) The placenta lies partly in the lower segment but its lower edge does not reach the internal os.

Type II: (Marginal) The lower edge reaches the os but does not cover it.

Type III: The placenta completely covers the os when that is closed, but not when it is widely dilated.

Type IV: The placenta covers the os even when it is widely dilated.

(Types III and IV were formerly described together as the central type.)

Clinical features

Whenever the uterus contracts strongly enough to stretch the lower uterine segment a low-lying placenta will be partly separated and bleed. This usually (but not always) occurs during pregnancy, but severe bleeding is inevitable during labour.

The bleeding is unrelated to general activity, although it may follow vaginal examination or coitus. It is painless, and often recurs. Dangerous bleeding during labour is followed by the usual signs of shock and anaemia. Unless the maternal blood pressure falls severely the fetal heart sounds are usually present.

Because the placenta occupies the lower uterine segment the fetal head cannot engage, and there may be a malpresentation.

Diagnosis

During pregnancy the differential diagnosis includes abruptio placentae cervical erosion, polyp and carcinoma. It is safe to pass a speculum to inspect the cervix, but unless an erosion is seen to be bleeding its discovery should never be taken to exclude placenta praevia. It must be added that in a number of cases of slight haemorrhage during pregnancy no cause is ever found, but the diagnosis of placenta praevia is so important that no case can be lightly dismissed.

Ultrasonic examination will nearly always show the position of the placenta. However, if ultrasonic examination made for some other reason in early pregnancy suggests that the placenta is low-lying, this conclusion is not always reliable at that stage, and it must be confirmed by repeating the examination in late pregnancy.

Clinical methods of diagnosis may be inconclusive unless a finger is passed through the cervix but *this examination is dangerous and may cause furious bleeding* if a placenta praevia is present. It should therefore never be done unless the diagnosis is otherwise uncertain, and then only with the patient anaesthetized in the operating theatre with all preparations made for treatment, including blood transfusion and Caesarean section. This investigation can usually be postponed until the fetus is mature enough to survive delivery.

Treatment

If bleeding occurs during pregnancy the patient is admitted to hospital. If bleeding is slight she is kept at rest and ultrasonic investigation is made. In nearly every case the position of the placenta is certainly determined. Only if this, and perhaps the fact that the head is engaged, proves that the placenta is not in the lower segment is she allowed to leave. In the few cases in which the diagnosis is uncertain the patient is kept at rest until about the 38th week, when a vaginal examination is made in the theatre.

If a placenta praevia is certainly demonstrated Caesarean section is the treatment for all except Type I cases. This avoids the haemorrhage which is otherwise inevitable during vaginal delivery. In Type I cases the membranes are ruptured and this allows the presenting part to descend and compress the lower edge of the placenta and so to control bleeding during labour. If no placenta is felt on vaginal examination it is still wise to rupture the membranes, as an extremely lateral placenta may be just out of reach of the finger.

In a few cases in spite of rest in hospital, or in emergency admissions, severe bleeding occurs. The treatment is Caesarean section as soon as any shock has been treated by blood transfusion. This should still be done even if the fetus is dead.

SPONTANEOUS PREMATURE LABOUR

This may occur with multiple pregnancy, hydramnios, sometimes if the fetus is abnormal, if the membranes rupture prematurely, and after fetal death. There is a tendency for premature labour to occur if the mother smokes heavily or has urinary tract infection. In many of these cases the fetus is also light-for-dates.

PREMATURE RUPTURE OF THE MEMBRANES

This may occur when the cervix is incompetent (p. 47), in cases of overdistension of the uterus by twins or hydramnios, or without explanation. Strong uterine action usually follows within a few days and the fetus is expelled; its hope of survival depends on its maturity. Sometimes labour does not occur for a few weeks. Liquor continues to escape and there is a risk of bacteria invading the uterus and causing fetal infection. To avoid this risk, if the fetus is large enough to have a good hope of survival (34 weeks) is best to stimulate uterine contractions with an oxytocic drip. If, however, the fetus is thought to be too small to survive, uterine action may be inhibited by a slow intravenous infusion of a β sympathetico-mimetic drug such as isoxsuprine or Ritodrine. Ritodrine is infused at 50 μg/minute in a 5 per cent solution of glucose in water, increasing the rate until contractions are inhibited, or a dose rate of 400 μg/minute has been reached. Antibiotics such as ampicillin may be given to prevent infection, but with uncertain benefit. Dexamethasone 4 mg 6 hourly for 2 days may also be given to the mother by intramuscular injection with the hope of preventing respiratory distress syndrome (p. 162). It should not be given if the mother is hypertensive.

POSTMATURITY

In about 10 per cent of pregnancies labour does not start until the 42nd week or later. The perinatal mortality is increased by about 1 per cent. The fetal head is larger and moulds less easily, and in a few of the cases there is placental insufficiency. Diagnosis is often doubtful. If the dates are uncertain the rate of uterine growth and the date of quickening are rough guides. An X-ray to show fetal ossific centres or ultrasonic measurement of the size of the fetal head may help.

Induction of labour is usually advised. However, if the head is not engaged and the cervix is unripe the risk of induction may outweigh the advantage. Labour can be induced with vaginal pessaries of prostaglandin E_2 in a suitable base. Alternatively, the membranes may be ruptured and a Syntocinon drip set up.

A careful watch is kept for any sign of fetal distress during labour. If this occurs in the first stage Caesarean section is required, and in the second stage forceps delivery. Because of this, these patients are safest in hospital.

INTRAUTERINE FETAL DEATH

Fetal death before labour may result from:

1. Placental separation or infarction.
2. Placental insufficiency due to hypertension or proteinuria or postmaturity.
3. Diabetes.
4. Obstruction to the cord vessels.
5. Fetal anaemia due to haemolytic disease.
6. Fetal abnormalities.
7. Syphilis.

The mother notices cessation of fetal movements; uterine growth ceases and the heart sounds cannot be heard.

If a dead fetus is retained it becomes macerated. The skin becomes discoloured and peels, and the tissues and ligaments soften. Overlapping of the skull bones can be seen on radiological examination (*Spalding's sign*), and gas may also be seen in large fetal vessels (*Roberts' sign*).

There is no immediate maternal risk; most patients go into labour spontaneously. Rupture of the membranes is dangerous as bacteria can then invade the uterus. Labour usually follows vaginal insertion of pessaries of PGE_2. If this is ineffective an oxytocin infusion may be tried or the injection of a hypertonic solution of urea through the abdominal wall into the amniotic cavity. There is a very small risk of hypofibrinogenaemia (p. 117), but only 3–4 weeks after fetal death.

ABNORMALITIES OF THE GENITAL TRACT COMPLICATING PREGNANCY AND LABOUR

Vulval varices.
Vulval varices (varicose veins) cause discomfort on standing

and occasionally rupture and cause a vulval haematoma during labour. Injection or surgical treatment is not advised as they usually shrink after delivery.

Vaginal discharge

Infection with *Candida albicans* (monilia) causes a thick white discharge with pruritus. If some of the discharge is placed in a drop of saline and examined with the microscope the filaments of the fungus are seen; it can also be cultured. The infection is treated with nystatin vaginal pessaries and also oral tablets to prevent possible reinfection from the bowel.

Infection with *Trichomonas vaginalis* causes a profuse purulent offensive discharge. Microscopical examination of a little of the discharge in a drop of saline shows the flagellated motile organisms, each about the size of a leukocyte. The treatment is to give metronidazole 200 mg three times daily by mouth for a week.

Previous perineal or vaginal repair

See p. 106.

Incarceration of the retroverted uterus

Uterine retroversion is present in 20 per cent of women and it seldom causes trouble in pregnancy. In a few cases the uterus does not rise up into the abdomen at the 12th week and continues to enlarge in the pelvis, causing retention of urine. The cervix is found to be displaced forwards with the body of the uterus behind it filling the pelvis. The full bladder must not be mistaken for the pregnant uterus. When a catheter is passed the uterus often rises up spontaneously as the bladder empties; if it does not do this it must be pushed up, under anaesthesia if necessary. No treatment is required for retroversion unless retention occurs.

Cervical erosions

These commonly occur during pregnancy. They may cause slight bleeding which can be confused with that due to placenta praevia but they require no treatment. They may also be found at a postnatal examination (p. 42).

Fibromyomata

Fibromyomata usually cause no difficulties during pregnancy or labour, but the following complications occasionally occur:

1. Most fibroids grow from the body of the uterus and are drawn up out of the pelvis as the uterus enlarges, but cervical fibroids are not drawn up and will obstruct labour.
2. Retention of urine is rare.
3. Abortion.
4. Malpresentation.
5. A fibroid may undergo acute necrosis (red degeneration), causing pain and fever. The symptoms subside in a few days without treatment.
6. Torsion of the uterus and mass of fibroids is very rare.
7. Infection and sloughing of the fibroid after delivery.
8. Postpartum haemorrhage, because the fibroid interferes with uterine retraction or because of sloughing.

Fibromyomata are felt as bosses on the wall of the uterus. On abdominal or vaginal examination they are not mobile like fetal parts. If the diagnosis is uncertain ultrasound may help. Caesarean section is seldom required except in uncommon cases of obstructed labour. Hysterectomy can be performed at the same time if required, but if myomectomy is proposed it is safer to postpone this until later.

Cervical carcinoma

Antenatal clinics are places where vaginal cytology can be done for women who would not otherwise attend. If the smear shows abnormal cells colposcopy should be performed. If a suspicious lesion is seen on coloposcopy or with the naked eye a biopsy should be taken at once, but otherwise the patient is followed carefully, repeating the examination after delivery.

Cervical carcinoma causes bleeding, and an ulcer or polypoid mass is found on examination with a speculum. If signs are present treatment is urgent.

Because treatment with caesium or radium cannot be effectively given while the uterus still contains the fetus and placenta, Wertheim's hysterectomy may be chosen for these difficult cases. In early pregnancy the operation is performed without emptying the uterus, but in late pregnancy if the fetus is viable it can first be delivered by a Caesarean incision.

Uterine malformations

When pregnancy occurs in a malformed uterus delivery is often uneventful but the following events sometimes occur:

1. The empty horn of a double uterus enlarges and forms a pelvic tumour which obstructs labour and makes Caesarean section necessary.
2. Abortion.
3. If pregnancy occurs in a rudimentary horn this may rupture at about the 16th week.
4. Postpartum haemorrhage.
5. A vaginal septum may be present and obstruct labour, but it is usually easy to divide this from below.

Ovarian cysts

These may be first discovered during pregnancy, labour or the puerperium. They may:

1. Obstruct labour if they remain in the pelvis.
2. Rupture.
3. Undergo torsion and cause acute abdominal pain and vomiting.

A cyst should be removed without much delay as it may be malignant. Operation can be postponed during the first 12 weeks to avoid the risk of miscarriage, and during the last month of pregnancy if the cyst is not below the presenting part. In all other cases a cyst should be removed at once. If a cyst obstructs labour it can seldom be pushed up out of the pelvis; Caesarean section is usually required to empty the uterus before dealing with the cyst which is impacted in the recto-vaginal pouch.

GENERAL DISORDERS COMPLICATING PREGNANCY

Anaemia

Retention of water during normal pregnancy causes an increase in plasma volume and a relative decrease in haemoglobin concentration. Values above 10.5 g per 100 ml can be accepted as normal.

Iron deficiency anaemia

This is common, especially in women who start pregnancy with poor iron reserves. The fetus and placenta contain 450 mg of iron at term, and blood loss and lactation each account for 200 mg. Diets poor in meat and vegetables often contain inadequate iron, and even good diets may only supply 15 mg daily, of which 2 mg is absorbed. Antenatal patients are usually given supplements of iron, such as ferrous fumarate 300 mg daily (with folic acid 0.3 mg daily).

In iron deficiency anaemia the red cell count, haemoglobin concentration, colour index, mean corpuscular haemoglobin content, and the serum iron concentration are all low. These tests need not all be done immediately, but if there is no response to oral iron in adequate doses (e.g., ferrous fumarate 600 mg daily), and it is certain that the patient is taking the tablets, complete investigation is essential. Other types of anaemia and pyelonephritis must be excluded. Iron can be given intravenously, but dangerous reactions sometimes occur. After a test dose of 1 ml, injections of 5 ml of Ferrivenin are given daily for seven days. If the patient is near term and the haemoglobin concentration is less than .10 g per 100 ml blood transfusion is required.

Megaloblastic anaemia

This is uncommon in Britain. It is due to folic acid deficiency. The red cells may be macrocytic, but examination of peripheral blood is not always conclusive; bone marrow puncture will show megaloblasts. Treatment is with folic acid, 5 mg three times daily.

Haemoglobinopathies

In the fetus most of the haemoglobin (HbF) has different amino-acid sequences in the polypeptide chains of the molecule from those in adult haemoglobin (HbA). HbF is gradually replaced by HbA in the first year after birth, but if the child has some disorder that prevents formation of HbA then HbF persists.

Sickle cell disease occurs in Negroes who inherit abnormal HbS from both parents. Few patients survive to the age of childbearing, but those who do have dangerous crises in pregnancy, and the fetus may die. Iron is useless in the treatment of the anaemia; maternal exchange transfusion may be needed.

With partial inheritance (sickle cell trait) the blood contains a mixture of HbS, HbA and HbF. Crises hardly ever occur.

Some patients inherit another abnormal haemoglobin HbC, and if they should inherit HbS as well, crises frequently occur during pregnancy.

Thalassaemia is an inherited abnormality, particularly of Mediterranean people, in which formation of the haemoglobin side-chains is defective, and the blood contains much HbF. Cases seen in pregnancy are usually of the minor variety; they may have anaemia and splenomegaly but are seldom dangerously ill.

Heart disease

The cardiac output rises during pregnancy to a maximum at about 28 weeks. This high output continues until term. During labour there is from time to time still greater increase in output. A normal heart easily meets these demands, but a diseased heart may fail.

Causes of heart disease during pregnancy

Rheumatic carditis is becoming less common, but still accounts for most of the cases. In prognosis the precise valvular lesions are less important than a history of failure, much cardiac enlargement or atrial fibrillation. Some cases of mitral stenosis may be treated by valvotomy during pregnancy, but it is preferable to operate at other times.

Congenital lesions now account for over 10 per cent of cases. Interatrial or interventricular septal defects, pulmonary stenosis, patent ductus and aortic coarctation usually do well. Patients with lesions which have not been corrected surgically and those with cyanosis seldom become pregnant, but the prognosis is then serious.

Coronary arterial disease is hardly ever seen during pregnancy.

Classification and prognosis

In the past these patients were often graded as below, but today this classification is seldom used.

I: No symptoms during ordinary activity.
II: Slight limitation of ordinary activity.
III: Restriction of activity, but comfortable at rest.
IV: Dyspnoea even at rest.

The mortality may reach 10 per cent in patients with heart failure, but it is very low in the others. The prognosis is worse with increasing age, pulmonary hypertension or congestion, gross cardiac enlargement or fibrillation. Reactivation of recent acute carditis may occur, or superadded bacterial endocarditis.

Diagnosis

Diagnosis may be difficult as breathlessness and slight oedema of the ankles occur in normal pregnancy. Although soft systolic murmurs may be heard in normal pregnancy, any harsh systolic or any diastolic murmur is significant. Minor alteration in the axis of the heart changes the ECG and radiological appearance slightly, but not enough to mimic serious disease.

Management

If a patient gets through pregnancy without heart failure she is likely to have a safe delivery.

During pregnancy she needs more rest, with help in the house, and often admission to hospital for rest after the 30th week. Adverse factors are anaemia, respiratory infection, and hypertension due to pre-eclampsia. Cardiac failure may appear as acute pulmonary oedema, especially in cases of tight mitral stenosis, or as slower congestive failure, especially in patients with large hearts or fibrillation. Digitalis or diuretics may be required.

Patients with valvular prostheses will be on oral anticoagulants. These are continued until shortly before delivery when heparin by injection is substituted.

Patients with valvular disease or congenital lesions may develop bacterial endocarditis, particularly in the puerperium.

Termination is seldom necessary. After the 12th week it is usually safer to continue; cardiac surgery is sometimes an alternative.

Delivery. There is no point in inducing labour before term. Vaginal delivery is best, and Caesarean section is only recommended for other obstetric complications. The second stage of labour is assisted with forceps or vacuum extraction under pudendal block, unless rapid easy progress is being made.

In the puerperium additional rest is given, but there should be free movement to avoid the risk of venous thrombosis. Breast feeding is allowed. Penicillin is given during labour and for a few days afterwards to prevent bacterial endocarditis. At the postnatal examination clear advice should be given about aftercare and family limitation (including sterilization in some cases). Dangers should neither be left unexplained nor exaggerated.

Pulmonary disease

Pulmonary tuberculosis

Active disease is found in less than 0.1 per cent of pregnant women in Britain, and routine radiology of the chest is hardly justified except for immigrants or for cases with clinical suspicion. Neither pregnancy nor labour has any adverse effect on the disease, provided that proper treatment is given. Rare cases of reactivation after delivery are related to increased domestic work and strain.

In active cases the usual chemotherapy is given. Prophylactic chemotherapy may also be given to patients whose disease has been inactive for less than two years. In active cases breast feeding is forbidden and the child must be separated from the mother until B.C.G. vaccination has caused Mantoux conversion, usually after six weeks.

Other pulmonary diseases

These are treated as in non-pregnant women. For fear of adverse fetal effects adrenal steroids should only be given to asthmatics when other treatment fails, and, for infection, tetracyclines are best avoided for fear of harming the fetus.

Glycosuria

Renal glycosuria of pregnancy

During pregnancy the blood flow through the renal glomeruli is increased and more glucose leaves the blood. Normally the tubules reabsorb all this unless the blood sugar level exceeds the renal threshold (10 mmol/l), but sometimes so much sugar leaves the glomeruli that tubular absorption cannot keep pace, and glucose appears in the urine when the blood sugar level is not raised. This is harmless, but must be distinguished from diabetes by a glucose tolerance curve.

Diabetes

This may first appear or first be discovered during pregnancy. A few women only show abnormal glucose tolerance curves during pregnancy (gestational diabetes). Some patients, including those with a family history, are particularly at risk (potential diabetes), and there may be a preceding history of the birth of abnormally large infants, hydramnios or unexplained stillbirths.

Provided that she is properly supervised the risk to a diabetic woman during pregnancy and labour is small, except in rare cases with retinitis or diabetic glomerulosclerosis. Her insulin requirements usually increase. Control is more difficult, especially in cases with renal glycosuria when sugar is lost in the urine and urine tests do not reflect the blood sugar level. Control may also be difficult if labour is prolonged or anaesthesia is required. After delivery the increased insulin needs fall sharply. The infants are often large (5 kg or more at term) so that labour may be more difficult. Hypertension, pyelonephritis, hydramnios and vaginitis caused by candida are other complications.

Even with modern treatment the perinatal mortality is still about 10 per cent. Intrauterine death may occur during the last month, or if the infant is delivered prematurely to avoid this risk it may die of hyaline membrane disease (p. 162). The incidence of fetal abnormalities is raised.

The cause of intrauterine death in diabetes is uncertain. With high but fluctuating material blood glucose levels the fetal levels will also vary, and the fetal pancreas secretes an excess of insulin, which does not cross the placenta. It has been suggested that this excess of insulin may cause episodes of severe fetal hypoglycaemia.

Management. The fetal results depend chiefly on the degree of success in controlling the diabetes. Measurement of the amount of glycosylated haemoglobin (HbA_1) in the blood may indicate how efective diabetic control has been during the preceding six weeks. Close co-operation between physician and obstetrician is essential. Patients are often admitted to hospital for stabilization, and usually from the 30th week onwards. Soluble insulin in divided doses is preferable to less frequent doses of long-acting insulin, and combinations of these may be needed. The fetus should be delivered before the 37th week unless diabetic control is completely satisfactory. An attempt at vaginal delivery by induction is often worthwhile, but Caesarean section is performed if any difficulty arises, or if the patient has had a previous section. In practice about half the patients require section. Although it is big the infant is lethargic and may have respiratory distress; it is often treated in an incubator for a time. Lactation often fails.

Acute fevers

In any severe febrile illness abortion or premature labour may occur. Most organisms do not pass the placental barrier, but those of smallpox, vaccinia, chickenpox, rubella, a few rare virus diseases, syphilis and toxoplasmosis can infect the fetus. Fetal infection with the virus of poliomyelitis occurs rarely. The treatment of acute fevers during pregnancy is the same as at other times.

Rubella

If the mother has rubella in the first 14 weeks of pregnancy the fetus may be infected, and congenital heart disease, cataract, deafness and mental retardation may result. Clinical diagnosis may be uncertain and investigation of antibody titre against rubella is useful. The titre does not rise until about the time the rash appears. If there is a raised titre soon after exposure to possible infection (and before the rash appears) this indicates previous infection and immunity to the disease. Conversely, a low initial titre and subsequent rise indicates present infection.

The virus may persist in the tissues of the child, and neonatal purpura or hepatomegaly may occur. With certain infection in the first trimester termination of pregnancy is justifiable.

Rubella vaccination of adolescent girls if universally applied, which at present it is not, should prevent rubella during pregnancy. Women found to be seronegative in the puerperium should be given the vaccine. Those who work in antenatal or neonatal units should also be vaccinated if they are seronegative.

Vaccination

Vaccination against smallpox should not be performed in the first trimester unless the patient has been directly exposed to the disease.

Poliomyelitis

Women appear to be more susceptible to infection during pregnancy, and they should be vaccinated unless this has already been done.

Malaria

Exacerbations may occur during pregnancy, and pyrimethamine 25 mg weekly should be given in malarious areas.

Toxoplasmosis

This is caused by a protozoon whose sexual cycle is completed in cats. The cats excrete oöcytes which may encyst in man and other species. Infection may only cause a transient maternal illness with lymphadenopathy, but it will cause encephalitis (which may be followed by cerebral calcification) and retinitis in the fetus. Maternal immunity develops, so that subsequent pregnancies are unaffected. The disease is unlikely to be diagnosed during pregnancy, although serological methods are now available.

Cytomegalovirus infection

The virus is a rare cause of fetal encephalitis and mental retardation.

Herpes virus Type II

The fetus may be infected during vaginal delivery from vesicular lesions of herpes genitalis, causing dangerous and widespread neonatal disease. To prevent this delivery should be by Caesarean section.

Venereal diseases

Gonorrhoea

Any purulent discharge, especially if there is urethritis, during pregnancy should be fully investigated. Both cervical and urethral cultures are taken (using charcoal swabs). If direct smears show Gram-negative intracellular diplococci, or if cultures on blood agar are positive, 2.4 g of procaine penicillin are injected, and then the bacteriological tests are repeated to confirm cure. Occasionally other antibiotics have to be used for resistant strains. If the infection is not eradicated before delivery there is a danger of infection of the infant's eyes (p. 163).

Syphilis

Every pregnant woman must have a serological test for syphilis. If this test is positive the result is confirmed with another of the serological tests and a treponemal immobilization test.

If the *Treponema pallida* is in the maternal blood it will invade the placenta and fetus. Late abortion, or premature delivery of a macerated fetus may occur, or the infant may be born alive with the disease. Living children may be underweight and show early clinical evidence of syphilis, but in other cases the disease only becomes evident after months or even years. The safest plan is to treat every pregnant woman who has or has had syphilis at any time. Ten daily intramuscular injections of 1 million units of procaine penicillin are given.

The serological reactions of the infant are tested at 4, 8 and 12 weeks. An initial positive result may only reflect that of the mother, but if the titre does not fall quickly the infant must be treated even if there are no clinical signs of disease.

Acute abdominal complications

Pregnancy may be complicated by any acute abdominal

catastrophe, such as appendicitis, cholecystitis or intestinal obstruction, and diagnosis is often difficult. Errors arise because the symptoms and signs of such complications are attributed to the pregnancy. In differential diagnosis extra-uterine pregnancy, abruptio placentae, uterine rupture, red degeneration of a fibroid, torsion of an ovarian cyst and pyelonephritis must be considered.

Acute appendicitis

This is a dangerous complication of pregnancy if it is undiagnosed and perforation occurs. The appendix may be high up and hidden by the uterus. If pyelonephritis is excluded by examination of the urine, and the site of maximum tenderness is separate from the uterus, laparotomy is performed through a lateral incision.

Jaundice in pregnancy

Jaundice during pregnancy is usually due to some intercurrent disease. The commonest cause is ordinary *infective hepatitis*; hepatitis transmitted from infected serum is now rare. The prognosis is good, and hepatic necrosis is a very rare sequel. Fetal involvement is rare.

Any of the numerous other causes of jaundice may complicate pregnancy, but the only ones worth mentioning are *gall-stones*, *drugs* (including chlorpromazine and fluothane) and *haemolysis* due to mismatched blood transfusion or infection with haemolytic organisms.

Jaundice very rarely occurs in eclampsia (p. 58). In *obstetric hepatosis* there is mild jaundice with intrahepatic cholestasis which recurs in the last trimester of successive pregnancies, often with pruritus. Patients on 'the pill' may show this. The prognosis is excellent.

'*Obstetric yellow atrophy*', i.e., fatal fatty degeneration and necrosis, may be a very rare specific disorder of pregnancy, but this is doubtful.

Common minor complications

Gingivitis and dental caries

Caries may progress during pregnancy and any cavities should be filled. If extraction is necessary and cannot be carried out under local anaesthesia a proper general anaesthetic should be given, not 'gas' in a dental chair.

Heartburn

This is due to relaxation of the cardiac orifice or to a hiatus hernia. Alkalis give some relief, and sleep may be easier if the patient does not lie flat.

Morning sickness

See p. 52.

Constipation

Laxatives such as senna are often needed.

Haemorrhoids

If these are painful an injection of proctocaine beneath them will give temporary relief.

Varicose veins

Varicose veins of the legs may get worse or appear for the first time in pregnancy. They tend to improve, at least partly, after delivery, and surgical treatment or injection are not usually advised during pregnancy. An elastic stocking is sometimes helpful.

Pruritus vulvae

This is may be caused by vaginal discharge. See p. 73.

Abdominal pruritus

Calamine lotion is more effective than antihistamines.

Acroparaesthesia (carpal tunnel syndrome)

Numbness and tingling in the hands during pregnancy may

be caused by compression of the median nerve by oedema in the carpal tunnel. Chlorothiazide may be tried but symptoms often persist until after delivery.

Nocturnal cramps

These are due to spasm of the muscles of the feet or legs, and are probably caused by circulatory changes. There is little to support the suggestion that they are due to calcium deficiency.

Supine hypotension

A few patients have hypotension and feel faint in late pregnancy if they lie flat, because the uterus compresses the large veins returning blood to the heart.

Miscellaneous conditions

Hyperthyroidism

This is treated with an antithyroid drug, and fetal goitre and cretinism is prevented by giving the mother thyroxine, which will cross the placenta. In small doses this will not affect the maternal hyperthyroidism. As an alternative thyroidectomy is possible during pregnancy.

Myasthenia gravis

The maternal condition is usually unaltered. Uterine action is normal. The infant may show transient myasthenia.

Chorea gravidarum

This is ordinary rheumatic chorea that has become reactivated during pregnancy. The prognosis is good.

Multiple sclerosis

Multiple sclerosis is unaffected by pregnancy, but the additional work of caring for the child may be detrimental. Termination has often been performed.

Cerebral thrombosis

The incidence is increased in pregnancy and the puerperium.

Epilepsy

Idiopathic epilepsy may become worse during pregnancy. The patient should continue her usual anti-epileptic drugs. If sodium valproate or carbamazepine are effective they are preferable to phenytoin, as there is a slight risk of fetal abnormality with the latter.

Otosclerosis

Otosclerosis is made worse by pregnancy.

Herpes gestationis

This is a rare skin disorder which recurs in successive pregnancies, with widespread erythematous and vesicular lesions.

Malignant disease

Most cases of malignant disease are unaffected by pregnancy. For cervical cancer see p. 74. Cancer of the breast may progress rapidly, especially during lactation. Termination may therefore be advised, and pregnancy is unwise for five years after apparently successful treatment.

Mental illness

See p. 134.

6

Abnormal labour

DELAY IN LABOUR

Delay during labour may be caused by:

1. Obstruction to delivery by:

Fetal factors	Malposition or malpresentation.
	Congenital malformation.
Maternal factors	Contracted pelvis.
	Pelvic tumours outside the genital tract.
	Abnormalities of the genital tract.
2. Inadequate expulsive forces	Weak uterine action and poor voluntary effort.
	Incoordinate uterine action.

Some of these factors will cause insuperable obstruction, but strong uterine action and good voluntary effort can overcome minor mechanical difficulties. On the other hand weak forces may fail to overcome even the normal resistance of the cervix and perineum. In modern obstetric practice poor uterine action is usually augmented by giving an oxytocic infusion.

'Rigidity of the cervix' is seldom a reality — if the cervix fails to dilate it is usually because the uterine contractions are abnormal or the presenting part cannot descend, not because there is anything wrong with the cervix. Resistance of the pelvic floor is easily overcome by general or local anaesthesia, which relaxes the muscles, or by episiotomy.

MALPOSITION

Occipito-posterior and Occipito-transverse position

At the onset of labour the head normally lies in the transverse diameter of the pelvis, or in one oblique diameter with the occiput anterior. The head flexes and descends and then the occiput rotates forwards (p. 29).

In about 15 per cent of cases the head lies in an oblique diameter with the occiput posterior at the onset of labour. In three-quarters of these cases spontaneous delivery occurs by one of two mechanisms:

1. The head flexes well and the occiput descends on to the pelvic floor. It then rotates forwards through three-eighths of a circle to the anterior position and is so delivered.
2. The occiput rotates back into the sacral hollow and then the head is delivered in the persistent occipito-posterior position (with the face applied to the pubis). The larger occipito-frontal diameter must sweep over the perineum (Fig. 14).

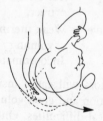

Fig. 14. Spontaneous delivery face to pubis.

In about a quarter of cases of occipito-posterior position difficulty arises. If the uterine contractions are not strong and the head remains extended, or if the pelvic cavity is relatively small, spontaneous rotation will fail. If the head remains extended the diameter of engagement is the larger occipito-frontal diameter (Fig. 8), and the anterior fontanelle presents. The wide occiput may be held up in the sacral bay and further extension of the head occurs.

In some cases the extended head is held up in the transverse pelvic diameter at the level of the ischial spines (*deep transverse arrest*). This may occur when the head was initially transverse, as well as in cases in which it was initially obliquely posterior.

If the head does not flex and descend on to the cervix less reflex stimulation occurs, so that uterine contractions are less efficient and labour is prolonged. The anterior lip of the cervix may also fail to be drawn up and become oedematous.

Diagnosis
The membranes often rupture early in labour. A slow first stage or lack of progress in the second stage should arouse suspicion. *Abdominal palpation*. Because the back of the fetus is situated more posteriorly the abdomen appears flatter, fetal limbs are felt anteriorly, and the heart sounds are heard well out in the flank. Engagement of the head is delayed because of the wider diameter of the extended head, and the occiput is felt at the same level as the sinciput. On *vaginal examination* during labour the larger anterior fontanelle presents and lies in front of the posterior fontanelle. If there is any doubt before forceps delivery the hand is passed up higher to ascertain the direction of the ear.

Management
If the first stage is prolonged additional analgesia may be needed. Adequate uterine activity must be maintained, if necessary by augmenting labour with an oxytocic infusion (p. 32). During the second stage time should be allowed for spontaneous descent and rotation of the head, but if after about an hour no progress is evident, or if the contractions are becoming weaker, or if fetal distress occurs, assistance is required. If the occiput is in the *transverse or obliquely posterior position* an anaesthetic (general or pudendal block) is given and episiotomy is performed. As alternatives:

1. A hand is passed into the vagina and the head is rotated to bring the occiput to the front. The shoulder is pushed round at the same time with the other hand on the abdo-

men. The head should not be displaced out of the pelvis unless rotation otherwise fails. Delivery is completed with forceps.

2. Rotation and extraction can be performed with Kielland's forceps (p. 149).

3. The vacuum extractor may be applied over the occiput, and with traction descent and rotation may occur (p. 149).

If the occiput is *directly posterior* and is very low it may be delivered with forceps without rotation, but if the occiput is higher or if there is any difficulty then rotation is required before application of the forceps.

MALPRESENTATIONS

Face presentation

Aetiology
This malpresentation is uncommon and occurs in 0.3 per cent of labours. *Primary extension* may occur before labour if, for unknown reasons, the fetus has increased tone in the extensor mucles of the neck. (After delivery the tone gradually becomes normal.) *Secondary extension* may occur during labour if the biparietal diameter is held up in the brim of a flat pelvis.

Diagnosis
This is rarely made before labour. In theory the prominent

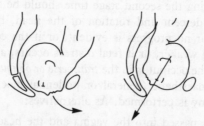

Fig. 15. Mento-anterior and mento-posterior presentation.

occiput is felt on the same side as the fetal back (Fig. 15). In practice, since the heart sounds may be heard through the front of the thorax in these cases, and on the same side as the limbs, the observer is often confused.

During labour the diagnosis is made on vaginal examination by feeling the facial structures. Late in labour oedema of the face makes this more difficult.

Mechanism

The diameters of engagement of the fully extended head measure the same as those of the fully flexed head (Fig. 8).

Mento-anterior position. With the chin anterior spontaneous delivery is to be expected. The head *extends* fully, the chin descends on to the pelvic floor and rotates anteriorly and is then born by *flexion* under the subpubic arch (Fig. 15).

Mento-posterior position. Spontaneous delivery may occur if the chin descends on to the pelvic floor and then undergoes long rotation to the front. If rotation fails impaction occurs because the head is already fully extended and therefore cannot be delivered under the subpubic arch (Fig. 15).

Management

Vaginal delivery usually occurs; Caesarean section is only required if there is pelvic contraction.

Mento-anterior position. Spontaneous delivery is expected. Forceps can be applied without correcting the position if there is delay.

Mento-posterior position. Impaction must not be allowed to occur. If spontaneous rotation does not occur after a short time in the second stage an anaesthetic is given, the chin is manually rotated to the front and delivery is completed with forceps. In very rare cases of impaction with a dead fetus craniotomy would be performed.

After delivery the face appears swollen and discoloured, but soon recovers.

Brow presentation

Aetiology

This malpresentation is uncommon and occurs in 0.2 per cent of labours. The causes are the same as those of face presentation, with one additional type of secondary extension. In this a head in the occipito-posterior position becomes extended still further if the occiput is held up in the sacral bay. This occurs in the pelvic cavity and only with a relatively small head.

Mechanism

Since the mentovertical diameter of 13.3 cm exceeds that of the widest pelvic diameter spontaneous delivery of a normal-sized head cannot occur unless it flexes or extends.

Diagnosis

This is seldom made before labour except when a high extended head is felt and an X-ray examination is made. During labour on vaginal examination the supraorbital ridges and the anterior fontanelle are felt.

Management

1. If a radiograph before labour shows that the head is extended nothing should be done until labour starts. Uterine contractions then often cause flexion (or rarely complete extension) of the head.
2. If the head remains extended above the brim when labour has been in progress for a time Caesarean section is performed, and always if there is pelvic contraction. Complicated vaginal manipulations such as internal version or correction of the position of the head are more dangerous.
3. Only in the case with a small head extended in the pelvic cavity mentioned above should vaginal delivery be attempted. Manual rotation of the occiput to the front and forceps delivery (or rotation and extraction with Kielland's forceps) is required — this is merely an overextended occipito-posterior presentation.

Breech presentation

Aetiology

Before the 30th week the fetal presentation is a matter of chance. Subsequently the fetus, by its kicking movements, usually adjusts its position to that in which it is best accommodated to the shape of the uterine cavity, so that in 97 per cent of cases the vertex presents at term. If the legs happen to be fully extended beside its trunk the fetus is unable to alter its position. In over 85 per cent of breech presentations the legs are extended, and this is the usual cause of persistence of this presentation.

In a *small* proportion of cases other factors are concerned:

1. The head cannot engage because of contraction of the pelvis, placenta praevia, a pelvic tumour, the presence of another fetus or hydrocephaly.
2. The fetal position is unstable because of a lax multiparous uterus or hydramnios.
3. The shape of the uterine cavity is abnormal, with a uni- or bicornuate uterus.

Types of breech presentation

The legs may be fully flexed at the hips and extended at the knees (frank breech), or the legs may be fully flexed at both hips and knees (complete breech). The arms are usually flexed before labour, but may become extended during labour.

Diagnosis

On *abdominal examination* the head, which is harder and rounder than the breech, is felt at the fundus, and is often mobile on the neck (ballottement). The fetal heart sounds are heard at a higher level than with a vertex presentation. On *vaginal examination* the coccyx, anus and scrotum can be felt, and with a flexed breech the feet present.

Mechanism

The extended breech engages easily in the pelvis. It descends on to the pelvic floor and the anterior buttock rotates forward so that the bitrochanteric diameter lies antero-posteriorly. Lateral flexion of the trunk now occurs so that the breech passes under the subpubic arch.

The flexed breech engages less readily, and there is some risk of prolapse of the cord as it fits less well into the pelvis.

The arms normally remain flexed while the trunk descends and is delivered. The aftercoming head enters the pelvic brim in the transverse diameter and then undergoes internal rotation, so that the trunk of the fetus (which has already been delivered) now turns with the back uppermost. The face appears at the vulva and the occiput finally sweeps over the perineum (Fig. 16).

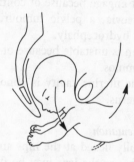

Fig. 16.   Delivery of aftercoming head.

Breech delivery is more dangerous for the fetus than vertex delivery. The risk in uncomplicated mature cases is about 2 per cent, but in complicated cases (prematurity, twins, prolapsed cord, contracted pelvis, etc.) the risk is very much higher. After delivery of the umbilicus, when the cord becomes compressed, delivery of the head must be completed within about 10 minutes; otherwise death from asphyxia would occur. The rapid delivery of the head, or the manipulation required to effect delivery, may cause a tentorial tear (p. 169), or less commonly injury to the cervical vertebrae or limbs.

Management

External version during pregnancy. Correction of the malpresentation by external abdominal manipulation is often possible if the breech can be disengaged from the pelvis. There is little point in this before the 35th week, as in so many cases spontaneous version occurs; after this time opinions differ about the wisdom of external version. In the past an anaesthetic was sometimes given to relax the abdominal muscles but, because of the risk of causing placental separation or premature labour by using too much vigour on the unresisting patient, anaesthesia is now not recommended, and even without it many obstetricians seldom attempt external version. Version is absolutely contraindicated if there is any history or risk of antepartum haemorrhage.

The place of Caesarean section. Because of the risk of vaginal breech delivery section should be performed when any difficulty is expected, or if the hope of subsequent pregnancy is reduced, as in the cases of:

1. Elderly primigravidae.
2. Patients with a history of infertility or obstetric disasters.
3. Patients with complications such as placenta praevia or prolapse of the cord.
4. Patients with small or android pelves. The pelvis should be carefully assessed clinically, and with an erect lateral X-ray if necessary, before attempting breech delivery.
5. If the fetus is unusually large or is judged to weigh less than 1800 g. Its size can be determined with ultra-sound.

Vaginal delivery may still be chosen for patients who have none of the problems just listed. In the first state of labour if the breech is not engaged the patient is kept in bed to minimize the risk of prolapse of the cord. In the second stage the breech usually descends steadily into the pelvis. It will not do so if there is disproportion or poor uterine action, and in either case Caesarean section is performed without delay.

In most cases the breech soon distends the perineum. At this stage a lateral episiotomy is performed under a pudendal block (previously inserted) or local infiltration. If the legs are flexed the feet are easily drawn down. If the legs are extended and there is delay, traction is made in the groin until the popliteal spaces are seen, when the feet can be disengaged. It is seldom, if ever, necessary to pass a hand into the uterus to push up and 'disimpact' the breech and 'bring down' extended legs.

If the arms remain flexed they will present as the trunk appears; traction should not be made at this stage as it may cause extension of the arms. If this should happen they are brought down by *Løvset's manoeuvre* (Fig. 17). The trunk is

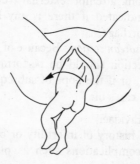

Fig. 17. Løvset's manoeuvre.

drawn downwards to bring the posterior shoulder into the hollow of the sacrum. The fetal trunk is then rotated (back uppermost) so that this shoulder becomes anterior, when it will present under the subpubic arch and can be brought down. The trunk is now rotated in the opposite direction (back upwards again) to bring down the second arm.

If there is any delay with the aftercoming head the safest method is to apply forceps, holding up the trunk and delivering the head slowly. As soon as the mouth appears the airway is cleared.

An anaesthetist should always be available for breech delivery in case any of these manipulations are needed.

Shoulder presentation

Aetiology

The commonest cause is multiparity, with a relaxed uterus and abdominal muscles. A second twin often lies transversely after delivery of the first, and sometimes does so in pregnancy. Rarer causes are subseptate (arcuate) malformation of the uterus, hydramnios, placenta praevia, contracted pelvis or pelvic tumour.

Diagnosis

This is obvious on abdominal examination. The possibility must not be forgotten during delivery of twins. On vaginal examination a presenting shoulder can be confusing, but the nearby ribs are usually obvious. If a hand prolapses it is distinguished from a foot by the absence of the heel and by the mobility of the thumb.

Course of labour

With a fetus of normal size obstruction will occur. Very rarely a small or dead fetus is delivered doubled up, but usually the membranes rupture early, the shoulder is driven down and the arm prolapses into the vagina, often with loops of cord. The uterus contracts down on the impacted fetal trunk, the fetus dies because the placenta is compressed, and eventually uterine rupture occurs.

Management

In multiparae external version is usually easy during pregnancy. The malpresentation tends to recur and these patients should be admitted to hospital from the 38th week so that frequent observation and correction is possible. Near term the presentation is corrected, an oxytocin drip is started, and when the uterus starts to contract well the membranes are ruptured.

In early labour correction by external version is sometimes still possible, but otherwise Caesarean section is best.

In neglected cases with the arm prolapsed it is possible to perform internal version and bring down a leg if the cervix is wide enough to admit the hand, provided that the uterus will relax under the anaesthetic, but if the fetus is alive Caesarean section gives better results. If the uterus is tightly contracted down the fetus is nearly always dead and internal version is highly dangerous as it may cause uterine rupture. Decapitation is then performed with sharp hook or embryotomy scissors. After division of the neck the trunk, is extracted by pulling on the arm and the head is delivered with forceps.

FETAL MALFORMATIONS

Figures for the incidence of congenital abnormalities mean little as the term is ill defined, but about 2 per cent of infants at birth have significant defects. Anencephaly, hydrocephaly and spina bifida account for a fifth of these cases, almost all fatal. If a patient has a child with a defect of the central nervous system in one pregnancy the chance of this occurring in a later pregnancy is increased, perhaps tenfold, but that still gives a 96 per cent probability of the child being normal in this respect. Antenatal diagnosis of open neural tube defects may be possible by amniocentesis (p. 155).

The following abnormalities may cause obstetric problems:

Hydrocephaly

If all patients are examined routinely with ultrasound in early pregnancy this may then be discovered and termination considered. Later in pregnancy the diagnosis is made by radiological or ultrasonic examination. The fetus often presents by the breech, and then the defect may be missed until labour. A severe degree of hydrocephaly will cause obstructed labour. Perforation is easy, and the head collapses so that spontaneous delivery may occur; otherwise forceps can be applied to it. If the obstruction is due to the aftercoming head of a breech a metal catheter can be passed up the spinal canal into the skull.

Anencephaly
Early diagnosis may be possible if routine early ultrasonic examination is made. If routine examination of maternal serum shows the presence of alpha-fetoprotein amniocentesis is performed and the liquor is tested for this substance. Ultrasonic or X-ray examination may be made in a case of hydramnios, or because the presentation is uncertain, and reveal the abnormality. If there is gross hydramnios the membranes are ruptured, and in other cases labour may be induced with prostaglandin vaginal pessaries. Difficulty in the delivery of the shoulders of a large previously undiagnosed anencephalic fetus can be overcome by cleidotomy and the use of a blunt hook in the axilla.

Other rare abnormalities
Other rare abnormalities that may cause obstruction include fetal ascites or tumour, and double monsters, but even with the last it is surprising how often spontaneous delivery occurs; otherwise Caesarean section or embryotomy is used without hesitation.

Rubella
See p. 82.

DISPROPORTION

Difficult labour may be due to disproportion between the size of the fetus and that of the pelvis. The outcome does not depend on the absolute measurements of the pelvis but on the relative size of the head, and good uterine action and moulding of the head will often overcome minor disproportion. Although pelvic abnormality is now uncommon in Britain abnormalities of the shape and size of the pelvis must be described.

Developmental variations in shape
The normal shape of the female pelvis is described as *gynaecoid*. The brim is almost circular except for the projection of

the promontory. If the brim is oval antero-posteriorly it is described as *anthropoid*, and if it is transversely oval as *platypelloid*. These variations are of no obstetric significance if the pelvic size is normal.

In about 20 per cent of women the pelvis has masculine characters (*android pelvis*). The brim is triangular in shape, but what is more important is that the subpubic arch is narrow, the ischial spines and side walls are closer together, and the sacrum is straighter than in the normal pelvis. The cavity and outlet of the pelvis are therefore reduced. Of course the outcome of labour depends on the size as well as on the shape of the pelvis, and in most cases vaginal delivery occurs, but in an android pelvis rotation of the head from the occipito-posterior or lateral position is more difficult, and the risk of breech delivery is increased.

Developmental variations in size
The pelvis may be small although its shape is normal (small gynaecoid or *generally contracted pelvis*). This is to be expected in small women, and if the fetus is proportionately small all is well. It also occurs in some women of normal stature, and in them the pelvis may be *funnel shaped*, with even more contraction at the outlet. This may be regarded as partial persistence of the condition found in the young child.

Other errors of development
There may be more or less than five sacral segments. The former (*high assimilation*) is disadvantageous as the pelvic cavity is longer.

The length and angulation of the coccyx vary greatly, but because it is mobile this is not important.

A rare abnormality is failure of development of the ala of the sacrum, so that the sacral bay on that side is reduced (*Naegele pelvis*).

Pelvic deformity due to disease of the bones
Severe *rickets* is now rare in infancy, but it can result in seri-

ous flattening of the pelvic brim. The rest of the pelvis is normal.

Gross pelvic deformity any also be caused by *fractures* or *achondroplasia*.

Deformities secondary to disease of the vertebrae or lower limbs
In *spondylolisthesis* the body of the last lumbar vertebra may project over the sacral promontory and obstruct the pelvic inlet. With severe lumbar *kyphoscoliosis*, which is often associated with a pendulous abdomen, pelvic deformity occurs.

If there is *paralysis, shortening or amputation of a limb* in childhood the pelvis is often asymmetrical, but normal delivery is usual.

Diagnosis

Before labour
Information about any previous labour is invaluable, including the result to the child and its weight, the duration of labour and the method of delivery.

At the 36th week of pregnancy the pelvis should be assessed by vaginal examination in every patient unless there has been a previous easy delivery of an average-size child. To assess the pelvic outlet and cavity the width of the subpubic arch, the distance between the ischial tuberosities, the distance between the ischial spines, and the curvature of the sacrum are noted. The brim cannot be reached unless the pelvis is severely contracted. If the sacral promontory can be felt its distance from the lower margin of the symphysis is measured with the finger, and subtraction of 1.3 cm from this diagonal conjugate will give the true conjugate (Fig. 7).

In primigravidae the head normally engages by the 37th week; in multigravidae the head often remains free until labour starts. In every case the way in which the head fits the brim should be assessed. This is done by pressing the head down, if necessary with the patient sitting or standing up.

If doubt about disproportion remains after clinical examination radiological pelvimetry is advised. From a lateral projection the shape of the sacrum and the position of the head can be determined, and the true conjugate can be measured. To avoid irradiation of the fetus other views are now seldom employed. The outlet can be assessed sufficiently accurately by digital examination.

During labour

If the head does not fit well the membranes may rupture early. Descent of the head may be arrested, but the observer may be deceived as to its true station if there is much moulding and excessive caput formation. If the head does not descend full cervical dilatation will not occur, and delay in dilatation may first draw attention to the abnormality.

Uterine action may become incoordinate; or the contractions may become more frequent and prolonged, ending in fetal death from placental compression and finally in rupture of the uterus.

Management

In cases in which it is judged that vaginal delivery of a living child is unlikely, and in cases in which the previous obstetric history justifies the operation, elective Caesarean section is performed.

In many cases, especially in primigravidae, the degree of disproportion is uncertain. In these cases a *trial labour* is conducted. The patient must be in a fully staffed obstetric unit because operative assistance may be needed at short notice. The spontaneous onset of labour is preferable, but if the pregnancy becomes postmature labour can be induced by insertion of vaginal pessaries of prostaglandin E_2 or by artificial rupture of the membranes. An oxytocic drip must be most carefully supervised.

When labour starts a careful watch is kept on progress and for any evidence of fetal distress. In some cases diagnosis of difficulty is only made when a partograph (p. 31) shows that there is delay in labour, and in spite of an oxytocic drip no progress is made.

Adequate relief of pain is essential; epidural anaesthesia is often useful.

There is no fixed duration of the trial; so long as regular progress continues and there is no fetal or maternal distress all is well. If, however, there is no progress during (say) three hours with good contractions after the membranes have ruptured, or if there is fetal distress, then the trial is abandoned. In most cases the cervix will not be fully dilated and lower segment Caesarean section is required.

If the cervix is fully dilated, and examination suggests that forceps delivery is possible this may be gently attempted under general anaesthesia in the theatre, so that Caesarean section can be performed at once if there is difficulty (*trial of forceps*).

Induction of labour before term is seldom, if ever, justified for cases of disproportion. It is occasionally recommended for a patient who has had a previous difficult vaginal delivery, if it is thought that a slight reduction in the size of the child will make a lot of difference — which is unlikely.

Treatment of cases first discovered in advanced labour
These cases may still be encountered in countries without modern obstetric services. If the fetus is alive lower segment Caesarean section is performed. Dehydration and ketosis must be treated first with intravenous fluids and glucose. Antibiotics are also given.

If the fetus is dead and the mother's pulse rate and temperature are rising craniotomy is performed if the head is fixed in the pelvis (p. 155). If the head is free above the brim Caesarean section, in spite of the risk of infection, may be safer.

In this country *symphysiotomy* is seldom performed, but in countries in which the patient may escape supervision in any subsequent pregnancy a Caesarean scar may be a grave danger, and this operation may have a place.

PELVIC TUMOURS AND LABOUR

Fibromyomata. See p. 74.

Cervical carcinoma. See p. 74.

Ovarian tumours. See p. 75.

ABNORMALITIES OF GENITAL TRACT AND LABOUR

Uterine malformations
See p. 75.

Cervical stenosis
After conization or amputation of the cervix stenosis is very rare. The thinned-out cervix may appear as a membrane over the head, when it can be incised; otherwise Caesarean section is required.

Previous colpoperineorrhaphy or repair of fistula
In most cases vaginal delivery is best after a generous episiotomy, but if stress incontinence or a difficult fistula has been cured then Caesarean section is wise.

ABNORMAL UTERINE ACTION

Each normal uterine contraction starts near the fundus and spreads downwards. The contractions of the thicker upper segment are stronger and persist longer than those of the lower segment, so that the latter becomes stretched and the cervix dilates. Between the contractions the uterine tone is low. At the height of the contraction the blood flow in the placenta is temporarily impeded, but intermittent squeezing of the placental blood spaces may be beneficial rather than harmful. Only if the contractions are unduly prolonged or frequent will the fetus suffer. There are several patterns of abnormal uterine action. In the past in Britain these were common and dangerous complications of labour. Since oxytocic infusions have been more fully used they have become less significant.

Hypotonic uterine inertia

The upper segment does not contract strongly enough to dilate the lower segment and cervix. The pains are weak and infrequent throughout labour. This may occur in a multigravida with a thin and overstretched uterus. Because the pelvic floor is relaxed spontaneous delivery often occurs, but there is a risk of postpartum haemorrhage.

Incoordinate uterine action

This was formerly a common complication of labour, especially if there was some mechanical difficulty such as an occipito-posterior position or a minor degree of disproportion. The contractions were described as incoordinate because they were irregular in frequency, duration and strength, and the upper uterine segment did not dominate the lower segment, so that cervical dilatation was slow. Many patients became distressed, and it was said that the disorder was caused by fear or emotional factors; but the chief reason for the distress was that the women were in pain for a long time without making any progress.

While incoordinate action may still occur, in modern practice with epidural anaesthesia and oxytocic infusion (see p. 32) most of the patients reach full dilatation and vaginal delivery, perhaps assisted with the forceps or ventouse. However, if the partograph shows no progress after rupturing the membranes and using oxytocin, or if there is any evidence of fetal distress, Caesarean section is performed without hesitation during the first stage of labour.

If labour is prolonged for any cause, dehydration and ketosis can occur, the risk of bacterial invasion is increased, operative delivery may be required, and postpartum haemorrhage is possible. Fetal distress occurs, and even fetal death in neglected cases. Intrauterine infection of a living fetus can occur, or invasion of a dead one by anaerobic organisms.

Prolonged labour should be recognized and treated with an oxytocic infusion, and Caesarean section if necessary, before this dangerous stage is reached. Fetal monitoring is invaluable and epidural anaesthesia often helpful. The urinary output is measured and the urine tested for ketone bodies. Dehydration and ketosis are treated with intravenous glucose infusions.

Constriction ring
In extremely rare cases there is a persisting and localized ring of spasm in the uterus (to be distinguished from the retraction ring of Bandl, see p. 22). It may occur around the neck of the fetus and obstruct delivery, or cause retention of the placenta in the third stage (*Hour-glass constriction*). It may follow intrauterine manipulations or the use of oxytocic drugs.

If the ring is encountered during attempted vaginal delivery or manual removal of the placenta it may relax with fluothane anaesthesia, or after inhalation of amyl nitrite 0.7 ml.

Cervical dystocia
This term is used when it is thought that obstruction to delivery is due to the cervix itself. If the cervix fails to dilate the usual reason is that uterine action is abnormal, or that something is preventing the presenting part from descending. However, stenosis may be the result of operations or carcinoma, and very rarely occurs without evident reason. If the cervix does not dilate Caesarean section is usually required; only if the cervix form a thin membrane in front of the head is it safe to incise it.

Obstructed labour
Although this is now rare in Britain, in some developing countries this very dangerous condition is still seen. If obstruction to delivery occurs from one of the causes given on p. 89 the pattern of uterine action alters. Vigorous contractions cause excessive retraction and thickening of the upper uterine seg-

ment and abnormal thinning of the lower segment, so that Bandl's retraction ring is accentuated and is so high up that it can be felt abdominally. The pains occur at shorter intervals and each lasts longer, so that they become almost continuous. Placental compression causes fetal death. With maternal exhaustion the pulse rate and temperature rise, and there is often dehydration and ketosis. Particularly in primigravidae there may be a period of incoordinate uterine action or inertia, but this is only a temporary respite. Eventually the uterus becomes tightly moulded over its contents and finally ruptures (p. 120). Before rupture the physical signs depend on the cause of obstruction, but there is usually a very large caput over a fixed presenting part, and the cervix and vagina are oedematous.

Immediate action is required to prevent uterine rupture Morphine 15 mg or a general anaesthetic is given to reduce the force of the contractions, and intravenous glucose solution may be required if there is dehydration and ketosis. If the child is normal and still alive Caesarean section is best, but if the child is dead vaginal delivery is sometimes chosen, although nothing should be done which will increase the risk of uterine rupture. For example, a hydrocephalic head can easily be perforated, but Caesarean section may be safer than craniotomy for a normal head impacted above the brim. Internal version is especially dangerous; decapitation is safer for an impacted shoulder presentation.

MULTIPLE PREGNANCY

Twins occur in about 1 in 80 pregnancies, triplets in 1 in 8000 and quadruplets in 1 in 500 000. There is often a family history of twins. Multiple pregnancy may follow induction of ovulation.

Uniovular twins arise by division of a single fertilized ovum. The twins are of the same sex and often remarkably alike. If the division is very early there are two placentae and sets of membranes, but usually there is a common placenta and chorion, with two amnions. Incomplete division gives rise to various rare forms of conjoined twins. An excess of liquor in one sac is common.

Binovular twins are three times as common as uniovular twins. The fetuses are dissimilar and may be of opposite sex. There are two placentae (which may be adjacent but have no vascular anastomosis), two chorions and two amnions.

If one fetus dies early in pregnancy it is retained and compressed in the membranes of the survivor (*fetus papyraceus*).

Diagnosis

The uterus is usually larger than expected from the period of amenorrhoea. Very early diagnosis can be made by ultrasound when two or more gestation sacs are shown. On abdominal palpation two heads and a multiplicity of fetal parts are felt. Sometimes one head is deeply engaged in the pelvis and only felt on vaginal examination. Fetal heart sounds may be heard at widely separated points, and with different rates. Suspicion should be aroused in any case of hydramnios — which is in any case the chief differential diagnosis. The diagnosis of twins can also be proved by ultrasonic or radiological examination in late pregnancy.

Complications of pregnancy

Vomiting may be excessive in early pregnancy and later there is discomfort and breathlessness from overdistension. The incidence of pre-eclampsia and of postpartum haemorrhage is greatly increased, and that of anaemia, placenta praevia and abruptio placentae slightly increased. The usual treatment for any of these complications is given.

Labour may start prematurely, and because of this and the risk of pre-eclampsia patients are usually admitted to hospital for rest from the 32nd to the 37th week. After 38 weeks fetal distress during labour is common with the second twin, and because of this many obstetricians advise induction of labour at this time.

Labour with twins

Malpresentations are more common and uterine action may be less efficient than in single pregnancies, and as intervention is often required an anaesthetist should always be available. In most cases the first twin lies longitudinally and is delivered spontaneously. The uterine end of the cord is clamped before it is cut in case the circulation of the second twin communicates. After respiration of the first twin is established the abdomen is palpated, and if the second twin is lying transversely external version is performed, preferably to a breech, and the membranes of the second sac are ruptured. If delivery does not quickly result the second twin is extracted as a breech, or with the forceps or vacuum extractor if the vertex presents. A breech presentation is preferred as extraction is usually easy, whereas the application of forceps to a high head may be difficult. Because of the risk of postpartum haemorrhage the use of intravenous ergometrine (as described on p. 38) is recommended.

In very rare instances the aftercoming head of a first twin may lock with the forecoming head of a second. If the heads cannot be disengaged and the first twin is dead its neck should be divided and the head pushed up, so that the second twin can be safely delivered.

Fetal prognosis

The perinatal mortality with twins is increased. The average weight of a twin at term is less than that of a singleton; in addition labour may start before term, or labour may have to be induced for some complication. Intrauterine death of one twin may occur, and to the risks of pre-eclampsia, antepartum harmorrhage, malpresentations and delay in labour is added that of prolapse of the cord. The fetal prognosis is even worse with triplets and higher multiples, and for these Caesarean section is usual.

PROLAPSE OF THE CORD

This is only likely to occur when the presenting part does not fit the lower uterine segment well because the head is small, or because there is a malpresentation, a twin, or disproportion. With hydramnios or during artificial rupture of the membranes the cord may come down when a rush of liquor escapes.

The prolapsed loop of cord becomes compressed between the presenting part and the cervix or pelvic wall, and fetal death will result. The term *presentation of the cord* is used when the cord lies below the presenting part with intact membranes. It usually escapes a dangerous degree of compression until rupture of the membranes occurs.

Management

If the fetal heart can be heard or the cord is pulsating, treatment is urgent. If labour is in progress and the cervix is fully dilated (or nearly so) immediate delivery with forceps or by breech extraction is effected. If the cervix is not so widely dilated Caesarean section is best. While preparations for the operation are being made the patient is kept in the Trendelenburg (head-down) position, or, better still, the presenting part is pushed up with the fingers in the vagina to relieve the pressure on the cord.

If the fetal heart cannot be heard there is no urgency about delivery, but disproportion or a malpresentation should be excluded.

PROLAPSE OF A HAND

This may occur with shoulder presentations (p. 99).

It may also occur with a cephalic presentation. As soon as the cervix is fully dilated the patient is anaesthetized, the hand is pushed up above the head, and delivery is completed with forceps.

POSTPARTUM HAEMORRHAGE

Bleeding from the birth canal after delivery may be:

1. *Primary*, occurring soon after delivery.
   a. from the placental site
   b. from lacerations.
2. *Secondary*, including all cases occurring more than 24 hours after delivery.

Primary placental haemorrhage

This still is, and should not be, an occasional cause of maternal death. It occurs during the third stage of labour or soon after delivery of the placenta. It is arbitrarily defined as a loss of a more than 500 ml of blood.

Aetiology

1. *Uterine atony*. This heading will include most of the cases. If the uterus does not contract strongly enough the placenta may be partly or completely separated but then the uterine tone may be insufficient to compress the vessels and control the bleeding.

The placenta may also be partly separated by unwise manipulation of the fundus, and then bleeding will occur if the uterus is atonic.

Uterine atony may occur:

a. When the uterus is thin and inert in grand multiparae. Postpartum haemorrhage can recur in successive pregnancies.
b. After long labour from any cause.
c. With deep inhalation anaesthesia.
d. When the uterus has been overdistended with hydramnios or twins. With twins the placenta is also larger than normal.

2. *Abnormal adherence of the placenta*. The chorionic villi may penetrate through the decidua into the muscle so that the placenta is partly or wholly adherent (placenta accreta). Separation is incomplete and the placenta remains in the upper segment, preventing efficient uterine retraction. A cotyledon which is left behind will have the same effect.

3. *Antepartum haemorrhage*. In cases of placenta praevia the lower segment does not retract well to control bleeding from the placental site. In cases of abruptio placentae the damaged uterus may not contract well, and there may also be a coagulation disorder.

4. Rare *uterine causes* of bleeding include inversion (p. 128), hour-glass constriction with retention of the placenta (p. 108), double uterus if the placenta is attached to the septum, and fibromyomata which sometimes interfere with retraction.

5. *Coagulation disorders*. See p. 117.

Diagnosis

This is usually dreadfully obvious. If treatment is delayed or ineffective anaemia and circulatory failure cause pallor, sweating, a rapid pulse and falling blood pressure, and even air hunger. If the uterus is atonic some of the blood is retained within it, and the fundus may rise.

Treatment

Some cases will be prevented by proper management of the third stage. Grand multiparae, patients with twins and those with a history of postpartum haemorrhage should be delivered in hospital.

Immediate treatment will usually stop the bleeding, so that circulatory failure does not develop, and if transfusion is required it can follow the local treatment.

In exceptional cases the doctor is called to a patient who is severely collapsed. The danger is greater if the patient was previously anaemic, or if unsuccessful but painful attempts to express the placenta have been made. If the blood pressure falls the bleeding may almost stop, and such a patient needs resuscitation by immediate blood transfusion *before* any local manipulation.

Treatment to arrest the bleeding:

A. *If the placenta has separated*. (For signs of separation see p. 37). The fundus is massaged to stimulate a contraction, and ergometrine 0.5 mg is injected intravenously if that has not already been done. The placenta is then expelled from the lower uterine segment, either by the Brandt-Andrews method (p. 38) or by gentle pressure backwards and downwards on the contracted fundus. The uterus is *not* violently squeezed — it is only used as a 'piston' to expel the placenta.

If, after delivery of the placenta and injection of ergometrine, the uterus remains or becomes atonic and bleeding continues *bimanual compression* is performed. A hand is passed into the vagina and shaped into a fist and then placed in front of the uterus. The other hand, acting through the abdominal wall, compresses the uterus against the fist.

B. *If the placenta has not separated* treatment is more difficult and depends on the facilities available:

1. If an anaesthetist and blood transfusion are immediately available, as in hospital, *manual removal* of the placenta under anaesthesia is performed. The fingers are passed up along the cord to the placenta and then directed to its edge. Starting at the edge, and with the other hand on the abdomen as a guide, the placenta is completely separated and when it is completely free it is withdrawn. (Credé's method, in which the placenta is forced out of the upper segment by squeezing, often causes shock and should be abandoned.)

2. If facilities are poor, e.g., with a single attendant in a house, it is safer to give an intravenous injection of ergometrine 0.5 mg (or failing that an intramuscular injection of Syntometrine). This will cause a strong contraction which will either separate the placenta, when treatment continues as described under A (p. 114), or will compress the retained placenta and stop the bleeding for a time. In the second event the help of the so-called obstetric 'flying squad' can be summoned from the obstetric unit, and manual removal is performed when an anaesthetist and blood transfusion are available, best of all without removing the patient to hospital, as there is some risk of further bleeding in the ambulance.

If the contractions are still poor after delivery of the placenta bimanual compression is performed as described above.

Primary traumatic haemorrhage

Unnecessary blood loss can occur from a *perineal tear* or *episiotomy* if suturing is long delayed. Any bleeding point should be controlled by pressure or ligature.

With a deep *tear of the cervix or vaginal vault* dangerous bleeding may come from a branch of the uterine artery. Such a tear is more likely with forceps delivery or breech extraction, but can follow normal labour. If rapid bleeding continues when the placenta is completely delivered and the uterus is tightly contracted this is the likely cause. Suturing can be difficult without proper anaesthesia, instruments and assistance; to place the sutures the cervix must be properly exposed with a speculum and drawn down well. While things are being arranged the bleeding can be controlled with a pack or manual pressure.

Secondary postpartum haemorrhage

Causes

1. Retained placental tissue. Intermittent bleeding occurs from the time of delivery and may become heavy.
2. Infection and separation of a slough from the cervix, placental site or a Caesarean incision. There may be offensive lochia and fever, and the haemorrhage often occurs after the 10th day.

Treatment

If the bleeding is not heavy and there is infection, local interference is deferred while antibiotics are given. Ultrasonic examination will show retained placental tissue. If the bleeding is heavy, or in any case in which there is a possibility that placental tissue is retained, the uterus is explored under anaesthesia with sponge forceps. Often nothing but blood clot is found and then washing out the uterus with hot saline and an injection of ergometrine are usually effective; packing is undesirable unless bleeding recurs.

RETENTION OF THE PLACENTA WITHOUT HAEMORRHAGE

Retention of the placenta may be due to:

1. abnormal adhesion; or
2. spasm of the lower uterine segment, which is sometimes the result of using oxytocic drugs in the third stage.

Even if there is no bleeding the placenta should be delivered within the hour. One attempt at expression may be justified, but if that fails manual removal should be performed under anaesthesia. Very rarely indeed a placenta accreta may defy attempted manual removal. It is then best left in place; hysterectomy would only be justified if there was severe bleeding.

COAGULATION DISORDERS

Failure of blood coagulation occurs in some cases of abruptio placentae, of amniotic embolism (p. 123) and sometimes when a dead fetus is retained in the uterus for several weeks. Bleeding from wounds or from the uterus may occur. The explanation is uncertain. Thromboplastin may be released from the damaged placenta and decidua, or from the amniotic fluid. Fibrinogen is used up in forming any large retroplacental clot, and there may also be widespread minute fibrin deposits elsewhere. Secondary fibrinolytic reactions complicate the picture. When intravascular coagulation occurs activators in plasma convert plasminogen to plasmin, which dissolves fibrin. Degradation products from lysis of fibrin themselves interfere with clot formation. There is therefore a complex clinical and haematological picture. There is fibrinogenaemia and the platelet count falls. The hypofibrinogenaemia is relatively easily treated. A quick and rough test for deficiency is to mix equal volumes of blood and thrombin solution (50 units per ml). If no clot forms, or the clot disintegrates within 60 seconds, there is considerable deficiency. This is treated by intravenous injection of a double strength solution of dried plasma.

Blockage of pulmonary capillaries by microclots may be more important than bleeding in some cases. For such cases heparin has been given.

OBSTETRICAL INJURIES

Vulval haematoma

A large vulval haematoma may occur during labour from subcutaneous rupture of a blood vessel. This is very painful and may cause shock. It should be incised to turn out the clot and relieve the tension. If the bleeding vessel is found it is tied.

Perineal lacerations

Perineal tears are not always preventable, but attention to the details of delivery of the head and especially the shoulders given on p. 36 will minimize the risk. An episiotomy is always preferable to an irregular laceration, and is nearly always required for malpresentations and operative deliveries.

Degrees

Three degrees are described:

1. The tear only involves the skin of the posterior margin of the vaginal orifice.
2. The perineal body and posterior vaginal wall are also torn.
3. A complete tear extends still farther back to involve the external anal sphincter and (usually) the anal mucosa. If a third degree tear is not carefully repaired the patient is likely to have incontinence of flatus or fluid faeces.

Treatment

All perineal tears should be repaired without delay. Oedema soon makes the repair more difficult. A third degree tear is relatively uncommon, but this is a serious injury and it is wise to transfer the patient to hospital where there are good facilities for the repair. For any repair local infiltration with 1 per cent lignocaine should be used, unless the patient is already anaesthetized or has a pudendal block. Chromic catgut or Dexon can be used throughout (plain catgut is too transitory). Non-absorbable sutures are sometimes used for the perineal skin and removed on the fifth day. The points that matter are to make sure that the top of the vaginal tear (which may be very high up) is found and sutured, to avoid tension, and to secure accurate and correct apposition of the various parts. For a complete tear the structures are repaired in the following order:

1. Anal mucosa.
2. Anal sphincter.
3. Vaginal wall.
4. Perineal body.
5. Perineal skin.

For less severe injuries the first two steps are not required.

After a complete tear the bowels are confined for 4 or 5 days. For less severe injuries no special care of the bowel is required except to wash and dry the perineum after defaecation. A bidet is very convenient for this.

If a perineal tear becomes infected the stitches may have to be removed, and if it breaks down secondary suture is performed when the infection has abated.

Vaginal lacerations

With severe perineal lacerations the vagina is always involved. More serious injuries resulting in *vesico-vaginal* or *recto-vaginal fistulae* are rare in this country. They may be due to unskilful instrumentation, but are more often due to prolonged pressure from the presenting part in cases of obhypostructed labour which causes ischaemic necrosis. Sloughing occurs some days later. Rectal injuries may heal spontaneously, but *vesical* injuries practically never do and they require repair some weeks later.

Cervical lacerations

Minor tears are common but unimportant. Deep tears may cause severe bleeding (p. 116) and such a tear may extend up into the lower uterine segment. A large haematoma may form in the broad ligament. This will displace the uterus upwards and to the opposite side, and may be big enough to be felt abdominally. Even large broad ligament haematomata usually absorb unevenfully, although the patient may be so anaemic that transfusion is required. Drainage is only needed if infection occurs.

Rupture of the uterus

This dangerous accident is now rare in this country, and almost all cases are due to rupture of a Caesarean scar. In a *complete rupture* part of the whole of the fetus may be extruded into the peritoneal cavity, into which bleeding occurs. In an *incomplete rupture* the peritoneal coat remains intact, but a large haematoma may form in the broad ligament.

Aetiology

1. *Rupture of a scar.* Classical Caesarean section is now seldom performed; the scar is less secure than that of the lower segment operation and complete rupture may occur during pregnancy or labour.

Lower segment scars seldom rupture except during labour. They are relatively avascular and stretch slowly. The rupture is often incomplete and little bleeding occurs, so that shock is slight.

Scars from myomectomy or from perforation of the uterus at curettage very rarely rupture.

2. *Rupture during obstructed labour.* This is very dangerous, with a mortality of perhaps 25 per cent. It occurs to a

patient who is already exhausted and may be infected. The tear is often in the posterior wall and may be extensive and complete. The ragged edges bleed freely and severe shock occurs.

3. *Oxytocic drugs*, in excessive doses will cause rupture.

4. *Obstetric operations.* Rupture can occur during such procedures as internal version and craniotomy, which are now rarely performed, and manual removal of the placenta. If the fetus is forcibly pulled through the incompletely dilated cervix that may be torn and the tear may extend up into the lower segment.

5. *Spontaneous rupture* occurs very rarely during labour in grand multiparae.

Clinical features

Rupture of a Caesarean scar is often 'silent' and diagnosis is therefore difficult. With an incomplete rupture symptoms are slight and consist only of lower abdominal pain between contractions, tenderness over the scar (if that is palpable in the abdomen) and sometimes a little vaginal bleeding. Shock only occurs if there is much internal bleeding or if the tear becomes complete. If the scar is adherent to the bladder that may also be torn and haematuria occurs. If there is serious doubt laparotomy and repetition of the section is wise.

In cases of rupture during obstructed labour the patient will be severely shocked. She may describe a sudden more severe pain with something 'giving way'. The history of the labour and the situation of the fetus will suggest obstruction. If the fetus is free in the peritoneal cavity it may be felt unusually easily. The fetal heart sounds will be absent. On vaginal examination the presenting part may not now be reached at all.

After vaginal delivery in which rupture is a possibility a careful examination of the lower segment under anaesthesia is made.

Treatment

Shock will demand blood transfusion. At laparotomy the fetus and placenta are removed. *Scar rupture* can usually be sutured after excision of the edges, but if the patient already has children sterilization is also performed. Hysterectomy is an alternative, especially for rupture of a classical scar. *Traumatic ruptures* are often extensive, ragged and infected, and hysterectomy may be unavoidable, but those who practise in undeveloped countries often recommend suture and sterilization. Antibiotics are given, and subsequent peritonitis and ileus are to be expected. A *cervical tear* which has extended upwards without reaching the peritoneum may sometimes be treated by packing.

Acute inversion of the uterus

This rare accident may occur spontaneously, or from pressure on the fundus or traction on the cord wrongly applied when the uterus is not contracting. The fundus, sometimes with the placenta still attached, appears at the vulva or is felt in the vagina, and the uterus cannot be felt in the abdomen. Shock occurs from traction on the appendages which are drawn down into the inverted uterus, and from constriction of the uterus itself by the cervix.

Treatment

Inversion should immediately be replaced under general anaesthesia. If replacement is delayed shock increases and replacement becomes more difficult. Immediate replacement by vaginal manipulation is usually easy, and 'hydrostatic replacement' with the pressure of water from a douche has been recommended. With immediate replacement neither fatal shock nor chronic inversion should be seen.

Maternal nerve injuries

Foot-drop due to paralysis of the dorsiflexor muscles with anaesthesia on the outer side of the foot may follow delivery. This may be due to:

1. Pressure on the lumbosacral cord at the pelvic brim during labour.

2. Prolapse of an intervertebral disk during labour.
3. Pressure on the lateral popliteal nerve from a leg support.

The prognosis is good, although recovery may take six months.

SHOCK IN OBSTETRICS

Acute circulatory failure during or soon after labour or abortion may be due to:

1. *Haemorrhage*, ante- or postpartum.
2. *Trauma*. Any misapplied violence during operative delivery or delivery of the placenta will cause shock. More serious shock follows uterine rupture or inversion. Long labour, with dehydration and ketosis, may precede any of these complications and cause 'exhaustion' — which may include both neurigenic and cortical factors.
3. *Anoxia during anaesthesia.*
4. *Undiagnosed cardiac lesions.*
5. *Amniotic embolism* is a very rare cause of sudden shock, dyspnoea and cyanosis during labour. During the height of a contraction a large volume of amniotic fluid enters a vein and death may be due to pulmonary oedema or widespread intravascular clotting. At autopsy the diagnosis is proven by finding amniotic squames or lanugo hairs in the lungs.
6. *Coagulation disorders* (p. 117).
7. *Incompatible blood transfusion.*
8. *Bacteraemic shock.* Endotoxins liberated from coliform or bacteroides organisms may cause vasoparalysis, with pooling of blood in the veins. The systemic blood pressure falls, but the central venous pressure may be normal unless there has also been blood loss, and the extremities may be warm. Tissue perfusion is inadequate, and later the skin becomes cold with cyanosis, and anuria and mental confusion occur. The choice of an antibiotic is difficult and will ultimately depend on the bacteria found. Gentamycin

3 mg/kg with clindamycin 20 mg/kg daily can be given orally, or chloramphenicol 30 mg/kg daily by injection in spite of its toxicity. An isoprenaline infusion (1 μg per minute) may be given.

Severe obstetric shock may be followed by pituitary necrosis (p. 133) or renal failure (p. 134).

7

Abnormal puerperium

PUERPERAL PYREXIA

Puerperal pyrexia has been defined as fever of 38° C or more arising *from any cause* within 14 days of labour or miscarriage. The causes include:

1. Genital tract infection (Puerperal sepsis).
2. Urinary tract infection (now the commonest cause).
3. Respiratory tract infection.
4. Thrombophlebitis.
5. Mastitis.
6. Any intercurrent illness.

Genital tract infection (puerperal sepsis)

Aetiology and pathology
Organisms enter the tissues through the placental site, or through cervical, vaginal or perineal lacerations. Infection usually occurs at the time of delivery, but may occur before delivery in a long labour, or may occur in the early puerperium. The following organisms may be responsible:

Aerobic haemolytic streptococci. These were the usual cause of the fatal epidemics of childbed fever of the past, but they are sensitive to antibiotics and are now less commonly found in the hospital environment. They are subdivided by serological methods; group A were formerly the most dangerous group, but today infections with group B are more common, and this group may also cause serious infection in the newborn child. Haemolytic streptococci are not found in the vagina before the onset of labour. They originate from another person with infection (puerperal or otherwise) and can survive on dust, blankets, etc., for a time, or can be carried in the throats of patients or attendants who may themselves have no illness.

Virulent haemolytic streptococci multiply in blood, causing haemolysis and breaking down of any clot. If resistance is insufficient there is very little tissue reaction and the organisms spread widely to cause local or general peritonitis, or cellulitis, or send showers of small infected particles of clot into the blood stream (septicaemia). The lochia is often inoffensive.

Anaerobic streptococci. The mode of spread of these organisms is uncertain; they are sometimes found in the vagina before labour. They can only gain a foothold in dead tissue or blood clot, which are likely to be present after much local injury. Suppurative foci are formed in the veins, causing spreading thrombophlebitis. The friable and partly liquefied clot breaks down to form comparatively large infected emboli (pyaemia), which cause metastatic abscesses in the lung and elsewhere.

Other streptococci seldom cause serious infection.

Staphylococcus aureus is commonly found in a hospital environment. It originates from some infected person, but survives for a time in dust, etc., and on the skin or in the nasopharynx of healthy carriers, including the noses, skin and umbilical stumps of infants. Fortunately, staphylococci usually only cause localized infection, but septicaemia can be very dangerous if the organisms are resistant to antibiotics, and then multiple metastatic abscesses occur.

Staphylococci also cause mastitis (p. 131) and ophthalmia neonatorum (p. 174).

Coliform bacteria. These organisms are constantly present on the perineum and often cause urinary tract infection, but sometimes also invade the genital tract. They usually cause localized endometrial infection with offensive lochia. They are a rare cause of shock due to liberation of endotoxins into the blood stream (p. 123).

Bacteroides. Organisms of this group occasionally cause puerperal or postabortal infection and endotoxic shock.

Clostridia. These organisms are rare but dangerous causes of uterine infection, more often after abortion than after labour. They come from the bowel and need dead tissue for anaerobic survival. Necrosis of the uterine wall, with peritonitis, septicaemia, severe toxaemia and haemolytic jaundice occurs, with high mortality. The mere discovery of a few clostridia in a mixed culture need cause no alarm — if they are invading they will obviously predominate in the culture.

Investigation of pyrexia after delivery

Every case should be fully investigated and all the causes listed on p. 125 should be considered. The history may help. With genital tract infection the fever usually starts on the 2nd or 3rd day, although severe streptococcal infection may give earlier fever. Genital tract infection is more common after operative delivery or manual removal of the placenta, but normal delivery does not exclude this possibility. Urinary tract infection may occur at any time. Infection of the breast is uncommon before the 7th day.

A full clinical examination is made, including general examination to exclude any intercurrent cause, and examination of the chest, abdomen, breasts, and legs. There are unlikely to be any conclusive symptoms or signs of genital or urinary tract infection at the onset, but the perineum should be examined and a pelvic examination made. In every case bacteriological investigation is required:

1. A high vaginal swab is taken for both aerobic and anaerobic bacterial culture, and all organisms are tested for sensitivity to antibiotics.
2. A midstream specimen of urine or one obtained by suprapubic bladder puncture is examined bacteriologically.
3. If there is high or recurrent fever a blood culture is made.

Clinical events

The following types of cases can be distinguished, although they obviously overlap to some extent:

1. Localized infection
   a. *Perineal infection*. If the sutures are removed resolution usually occurs rapidly, and further spread is rare.
   b. *Endometritis*. Often there are no symptoms or signs except fever of about 38.5° C. Sometimes the lochia is offensive (but not in streptococcal cases) and uterine involution may be delayed. Most cases resolve in a few days even without treatment, but with antibiotics resolution often occurs in 48 hours.

2. Spread to structures around the uterus
   The time when this occurs depends on the virulence of the organisms, but it is often after the 4th day. The fever and tachycardia of the initial endometritis increase, and there is lower abdominal pain. At this stage the pelvic cellular tissue and the adjacent peritoneum are both inflamed. Because of the *pelvic peritonitis* there is lower abdominal tenderness, and on vaginal examination any movement of the uterus causes pain. The peritonitis usually resolves, but sometimes an abscess forms which may point into the rectum or above the inguinal ligament.

   Pelvic cellulitis (Parametritis) also usually resolves, but sometimes takes several weeks to do so. An inflammatory induration is found on one or both sides of the cervix, fixing it firmly.

   Especially with anaerobic streptococcal infections widespread *thrombophlebitis* of the pelvic veins may occur, sometimes spreading downwards to the femoral vein or upwards to the iliac veins. There is a swollen 'white leg', and also infected emboli may be thrown off to cause repeated rigors and pyrexial episodes and metastatic lung abscesses.

   The infection may involve the uterine tubes, causing *salpingitis* and infertility.

3. Generalized peritonitis

When haemolytic streptococcal infections were prevalent and antibiotics were not available, spread to the general peritoneal cavity was disastrous, giving a mortality of 75 per cent. The pulse rate rose rapidly to 140 or more per minute, with fever of variable degree. Abdominal distention with little pain or guarding often occurred.

4. Septicaemia

This was also disastrous in the past but most organisms now respond well to antibiotics. The temperature is very high, swinging up to peaks of 40.5° C with rigors. Also see bacteraemic shock, p. 123.

Prevention

Anyone with a streptococcal or staphylococcal lesion (e.g., a sore throat or a paronychia) should not attend on labouring or lying-in women. Any patient with a puerperal or other significant infection must be isolated, and her room must be fumigated before further use by other patients.

Impervious masks must always be worn in the labour ward. Sterilized gloves must be worn for any pelvic examination. Proper care during vaginal examination is important, and such examinations should not be made unnecessarily. Catheterization is avoided whenever possible. If a midstream specimen is not satisfactory, suprapubic bladder puncture gives a better specimen for bacteriological purposes than catheterization.

Treatment

The immediate use of an appropriate antibiotic will prevent most of the events described above. If there is serious fear of a genital tract infection (e.g. with fever after criminal abortion or after long labour) treatment with ampicillin and metronidazole may be started at once, but in many cases the bacteriological report on the sensitivity of the organisms can be awaited so that the appropriate drug is used.

Local treatment is seldom required. The uterus should only be explored if the history of the case or bleeding suggests that placental tissue is retained. A pelvic abscess must be drained, or occasionally surgical treatment is required for a metastatic abscess.

For the rare clostridial infections antiserum is required as well as penicillin, and these are the only cases in which the desperate measure of hysterectomy might be seriously considered. Hyperbaric oxygen may be used.

Infection of the urinary tract

This is common in the early puerperium, either as a recurrence of an infection which was present during pregnancy, or as a result of catheterization and trauma to the bladder during labour. *E. coli* is the commonest organism found, but *Strep. faecalis*, *B. proteus* or mixed infections may be discovered. The genital tract may be invaded at the same time.

Clinical features
Often the only sign is mild fever, and there may be no urinary symptoms. The infection is usually confined to the lower urinary tract, but acute pyelonephritis occasionally occurs.

Diagnosis
Diagnosis rests on microscopical and bacterial examination of a midstream or suprapubic specimen of urine.

Treatment
Treatment will depend on the organisms found and their sensitivity, but most cases respond to sulphadimidine (2 g followed by 1 g 6-hourly), or to ampicillin (500 mg 6-hourly).

Abnormalities of the breast

Acute engorgement
On about the 4th day the breasts may become tense and painful because of hyperaemia and the onset of secretion of milk

into the acini. The tension within the fascial compartments interferes with the outflow of milk, which is the natural method of relief. Slight pyrexia may occur, but other possible causes of fever must be excluded. The breasts should be well supported. Manual expression or the use of an electric pump may be tried, but are often too painful.

Inhibition of lactation
Lactation can be suppressed with bromocriptine, 2.5 mg orally twice daily for 14 days. It inbibits the pituitary secretion of prolactin.

Cracked nipples
Small fissures may occur on the nipple or areola if the infant 'chews' too vigorously or for too long when there is insufficient milk. Cracks are acutely painful, and sometimes bleed, so that the infant may swallow and then vomit blood.

Treatment. Cracks should be prevented by careful supervision of the early feeds. The only effective treatment is to stop feeding from that breast for 24 to 48 hours, and to express the milk. Any local antiseptic application should not poison the baby, stick to the fissure or cause skin sensitization. Flavine in paraffin is recommended. If the fissure does not heal in this time breast feeding usually has to be abandoned.

Acute mastitis
This is due to invasion of the ducts by *Staphylococcus aureus*, which may be carried by healthy attendants or babies. Epidemics may occur in hospital. Organisms may also enter the superficial tissues through a cracked nipple, but this is not the usual entry.

Clinical features. Mastitis may occur at any time after the 4th day of the puerperium. Fever (40° C) and pain occur. A sector of the breast is hyperaemic, tense and tender. Axillary glands may be enlarged. If suppuration occurs a localized abscess may form and point, or spreading infection may cause widespread disorganization of the breast.

Treatment. The milk is cultured, and while the report on the sensitivity of the organisms is awaited antibiotic treatment may be started. In hospital staphylococci may be penicillin resistant, but the characteristics of the prevalent strain are often known. The breast is supported, feeding is stopped from that side, and the milk is expressed. If the skin shows brawny oedema, even without fluctuation, pus is likely to be present and an incision is made.

Galactocele
A small painless cyst may occur on one of the ducts near the areola. If it persists it is excised.

Carcinoma of the lactating breast
This is rare but lethal. A pre-existing cancer may progress rapidly, and termination of pregnancy may be advised on this account. Florid encephaloid cancer during lactation must not be mistaken for a breast abscess.

Secondary postpartum haemorrhage
See p. 116.

VENOUS THROMBOSIS

Thrombosis of superficial veins in the legs
This is common after delivery, especially if the veins are varicose. A tender segment is felt. Pulmonary embolism rarely occurs, so that anticoagulants are not used and ambulation is encouraged. Varicose veins may need subsequent surgical treatment.

Thrombosis of deep veins in the legs
This may occur at about the 7th day after delivery (and, rarely, during pregnancy), without any evidence of infection. It is commoner after Caesarean section than after vaginal

delivery. The calf veins are usually first involved. Venograms show that thrombosis of these veins may occur without symptoms, but there may be pain, swelling in the leg, pain on dorsiflexion of the foot, and a slight rise of temperature and pulse rate. In a few severe cases with spreading thrombosis and superadded vascular spasm the limb is white or blue. There are two dangers:

1. *Pulmonary embolism.* This often occurs without any previous complaint of pain or swelling in the legs. Any patient who has previously had deep vein thrombosis or a pulmonary embolus should be given anticoagulant treatment (in the form of subcutaneous heparin injections) throughout the antenatal period.
2. Permanent impairment of the circulation in the leg.

Treatment. Early ambulation after delivery reduces the risk of deep thrombosis. If it occurs anticoagulant drugs will certainly increase the rate of recovery of the limb, and may reduce the risk of embolism. Intravenous administration of heparin is started at once (10 000 units 8-hourly for 48 hours), and an oral anticoagulant such as warfarin sodium. An initial dose of 50 mg is given; the prothrombin time is measured and subsequent doses of oral anticoagulant (usually between 3 and 10 mg daily in divided doses) are adjusted to increase this two or three fold.

The leg should be rested for 2 or 3 days until the pain is less and the anticoagulants have begun their work, and then activity should gradually be restored. An elastic stocking may be used for a time.

Thrombosis of pelvic veins
Thrombosis of pelvic veins may be caused by infection (p. 128).

POSTPARTUM PITUITARY NECROSIS

This is a rare sequel of severe and prolonged shock, usually due to postpartum haemorrhage. Thrombosis of the vessels supplying the anterior lobe of the pituitary gland causes ischaemic necrosis. There is deficiency of prolactin and of gonadotrophic, corticotrophic and thyrotrophic hormones. Failure of lactation is followed by genital atrophy and amenorrhoea. The patient is lethargic, with anorexia, and a low basal metabolic rate. She usually gains weight. Treatment with thyroid and adrenal cortical hormones may give partial relief.

RENAL CORTICAL NECROSIS AND LOWER NEPHRON NECROSIS

These rare conditions, which may follow accidental antepartum haemorrhage or septic abortion, cause anuria after delivery. To circulatory failure and anaemia is added the effect of reflex spasm of the renal arterioles. In cases of bilateral renal cortical necrosis all the glomeruli and parts of all the tubules are killed by ischaemia. In lower nephron necrosis there is widespread damage to tubules, but many will recover.

In both cases anuria occurs, with a progressive rise in the blood urea concentration. If the case is one of cortical necrosis death is inevitable unless renal dialysis is performed. In tubular necrosis spontaneous diuresis and recovery may occur after about 10 days.

Treatment. Glucose solution is given intravenously, but the fluid intake must not exceed the loss by perspiration and sweating. If diuresis does not occur in a few days dialysis by the artificial kidney is required and possibly eventual renal transplantation.

MENTAL ILLNESS

During pregnancy and the puerperium women have to make adjustments to many new emotional experiences. Most women are ambivalent in their reactions. The wish for pregnancy and the desire to have children (whether determined by innate character or by imitation of other women) are counterbalanced by anxieties about labour, the unborn child, relations with her husband, and many practical domestic and economic problems. Minor symptoms, such as vomiting or insomnia, may be a reflection of these feelings. Kindness, understanding and wise counsel from doctors, midwives and relatives will assist in the adjustment, which most women make admirably.

Immediate contact of mother and baby after delivery, and breast feeding, may increase 'bonding', whereas separation during the early weeks because of illness of one or the other may have an adverse effect. If bonding does not occur, or if there are social problems, the risk of 'baby battering' or of maladjustment is increased.

Significant psychological illness occur in a few patients. Most of these have pre-existing instability and would react badly to any stress; pregnancy is not the specific cause of their mental illness.

Persistent insomnia, confusion, any obsession or hallucination, or any threat to the baby should be taken seriously, and expert advice sought. *Depression* may occur in early pregnancy, and is common as a transient attack of 'the weeps' in the early puerperium. More severe depression can be a serious puerperal illness with a real danger of suicide or infanticide. *Acute mania* is rare. *Schizophrenia* may recur or first appear after delivery. Prolonged puerperal fever used to be followed by toxic *'confusional insanity'*, but this is now rare.

Treatment of these conditions falls to the psychiatrist, but problems arise with the family and the care of the baby. Fortunately the prognosis is usually good, and certification is seldom required.

Termination of pregnancy

Firm psychiatric indications for termination only arise if the psychiatrist is unable to treat the patient by any other method, if spontaneous recovery is unlikely, or if any threat of suicide is real, but these indications are very often justifiably extended because of grave social problems. Sterilization may need consideration.

8

The fetus at risk in late pregnancy and during labour

Apart from mechanical problems during labour caused by malpresentations and disproportion, which may often be anticipated by antenatal care, some other cases of high fetal risk are foreseeable, and women with any of them should be cared for in fully equipped units with experienced staff.

Perinatal mortality increases when *maternal age* exceeds about 30 years, chiefly because of the more frequent need for operative delivery, and the increased incidence of hypertension and congenital malformations. The risk is also increased in women of *social classes IV and V*, because of poor nutrition and physique, premature labour and high parity, and sometimes because of lack of regular obstetric care.

Placental function may be impaired with *hypertension and proteinuria* caused by pre-eclampsia or essential hypertension, or (uncommonly) nephritis. With *urinary tract infection* the fetus is unlikely to die, but it may be both small-for-dates and born early. If the fetus survives an acute episode of *antepartum haemorrhage* the placenta may be left damaged. With *multiple pregnancies* one or more of the fetuses may be small because of placental inadequacy. In some cases of *postmaturity* placental insufficiency occurs.

If the mother *smokes heavily* the fetus tends to be small, especially if there is also hypertension. The reason is uncertain; it is more likely to be vascular spasm in the placental vessels than an increased blood level of carbon monoxide, although the latter occurs.

Haemolytic disease and *diabetes* are other conditions of fetal risk that can be recognized during pregnancy.

In the absence of placental insufficiency, if the fetus is born prematurely, whether spontaneously or by induction, it will be small; but only to the degree expected from the gestational age, and death before or during labour is uncommon. With placental insufficiency, however, the fetus tends to be light-for-dates and may die *in utero*.

During pregnancy warning of high fetal risk may be derived from the obstetric history, or by observing that the fetus is not growing normally, perhaps with the help of ultrasonic measurements. It may then be monitored during pregnancy by repeated placental function tests (p. 64), and also by observing whether it shows normal responses in its movements and heart rate (p. 18).

If the fetus is thought to be at risk the patient must be delivered in a fully-equipped obstetric unit, and when neonatal difficulties are anticipated she should be delivered in a unit with a full paediatric special-care facilities.

With all these conditions there is an increased incidence of fetal distress during labour, and to clinical vigilance it is desirable to add electronic monitoring of the fetal heart rate, with fetal blood sampling when appropriate. (See p. 33).

9

Haemolytic disease

Apart from the antigens of the ABO system red blood cells contain antigens of the rhesus system (so-called because they were first found in blood of rhesus monkeys). Every normal individual has 23 pairs of chromosomes in each cell. It is believed that one pair carries the rhesus genes, with three genes on each chromosome. Thus any one chromosome has C or c, D or d, and E or e, so that the pair of chromosomes will carry such combinations as CDe/cde, CDe/CDe, cDE/cde, cde/cde, CDe/cDE, etc. (Those listed include 99 per cent of combinations found in London women.) If an individual has the D gene on one or both chromosomes he is said to be rhesus positive, and rhesus negative if he has no D gene on either chromosome. If he has a D gene on both chromosomes he is homozygous for D and will transmit D to all his children, but if he has D on only one of the pair of chromosomes only half his children will inherit the D gene.

If Rh positive cells are introduced into the circulation of a Rh negative individual he will produce antibodies against the Rh antigen which the cells carry, and these antibodies will cause agglutination and haemolysis of the red cells. Reactions to antigens of this system other than D are very rare.

Rh immunization may occur because a transfusion of Rh positive cells has been given to a Rh negative woman, or because she has a Rh positive fetus in her uterus from which a few red cells have entered her circulation. If immunization occurs Rh antibodies are produced which cross the placental barrier and cause haemolysis of the Rh positive red cells of the fetus. During pregnancy very few fetal cells enter the maternal circulation, so that the fetus is usually unaffected in a first pregnancy, but at the time of the first delivery a large number of cells may enter the maternal circulation and cause sensitization. In a subsequent pregnancy even a very small transfusion of fetal cells will evoke the production of large amounts of antibodies, so that all subsequent Rh positive children that the mother carries are likely to be affected.

In Britain 15 per cent of persons are Rh negative. A Rh negative woman therefore has an 85 per cent chance of marrying a Rh positive husband, and as he has about a half chance of being homozygous it can be calculated that the expected incidence of Rh incompatibility is about 8 per cent, but in fact the fetus is affected in only about 0.5 per cent of the cases because the volume of fetal blood tranfused and the maternal reaction to antigen are variable, and because any fetal cells which are also ABO incompatible are agglutinated and may not induce Rh immunity reactions.

There are two types of Rh antibodies. 'Saline antibodies' agglutinate red cells suspended in saline, but are of little clinical importance. 'Albumin antibodies' agglutinate red cells suspended in a solution of albumin, and these cross the placenta; they can be detected by Coombs' antiglobulin test.

Effect on the fetus or newborn child

If the fetus is severely affected it becomes anaemic, and cardiac failure eventually causes generalized oedema, ascites and pleural effusions (*Hydrops fetalis*). Intrauterine death almost invariably occurs, between the 28th week and term. The placenta is large and oedematous, and all the primitive centres of red cell formation (liver, spleen, lymph glands, etc.) remain active (*Erythroblastosis fetalis*). The fetus, placenta and liquor amnii are bile stained.

In moderately severe cases the fetus is born alive, but deep jaundice soon appears (*Icterus gravis neonatorum*). While the fetus is in the uterus the placenta removes much of the excess bilirubin produced by destruction of red cells, but after birth haemolysis continues for a time and the liver is unable to con-jugate all the bilirubin. The liver may be enlarged. High levels of bilirubin in the blood (over 340 mmol/l) damage the basal nuclei of the brain (*Kernicterus*). Neck rigidity, nystagmus and twitching occur, and if the child survives there is spasticity or mental retardation.

In mild cases *haemolytic anaemia* occurs in the first fort-night, but jaundice is slight. Nucleated red cells are found in the blood.

Diagnosis

All antenatal patients must have their blood group determined and those that are Rh negative are also tested for Rh anti-bodies, both early in pregnancy and at the 30th and 36th weeks. Those with antibodies require frequent tests. Slight changes in antibody titre mean little, but high levels or sudden changes are danger signals. Amniocentesis may be necessary to assess the degree of fetal risk (see below).

The history of any previous pregnancies is always helpful. Sometimes the husband's blood is also examined to determine (if possible) his genetic pattern.

After delivery the child's blood group is determined and Coombs' antiglobulin test will show whether the red cells have been sensitized to antibody. The haemoglobin level is esti-mated and nucleated red cells may be counted.

Prevention

If an injection of anti-D globulin (100 μg intramuscularly) is given to a rhesus negative mother (who has not previously been immunized) within 48 hours of the birth of a rhesus positive baby most cases of rhesus immunization can be pre-vented. The globulin is obtained from the blood of another patient or volunteer who has been immunized. The number of fetal cells in the maternal blood after delivery can be roughly estimated by the Kleihauer method of staining a film, which distinguishes the cells with fetal haemoglobin. The risk of immunization is greater if the fetal cell count is high, and also if the fetal and maternal cells are ABO compatible. The globulin blocks the immunity reaction to D cells, but the mechanism is still uncertain; it is probably not due to simple elimination of D cells from the blood.

Treatment

Mild cases need no treatment, but in many cases the child requires an *exchange transfusion* after delivery, using Rh negative blood, to tide it over until the action of the maternal antibodies ceases. This is done not only to treat anaemia but also to prevent kernicterus. When the sensitized Rh positive cells are replaced the bilirubin level can rise no further, and the exchange also removes some bilirubin. Fresh blood is used at room temperature. After the apparatus has been washed out with a little heparin solution a fine polythene catheter is passed into the umbilical vein. A second catheter is inserted into the antecubital vein. Blood is withdrawn at a constant rate from one catheter, while donor blood is injected through the other at the same rate until a total of 150 ml per kg has been given. Repeated exchanges may be made if the bilirubin level rises dangerously.

In severe cases, and in those with a history of a previous intrauterine death, delivery at the 35th week or even earlier is sometimes advised to remove the fetus from the action of maternal antibodies. This will only give good results if expert care can be given to the premature baby, including repeated exchange transfusion if necessary.

The assessment of severity in a particular pregnancy is not always easy, and if the father's group is heterozygous it may even be uncertain whether the fetus is Rh positive. Spectro-photometric estimation of the bilirubin content of a sample of liquor amnii obtained with a needle through the abdominal wall will assist in determining whether haemolysis is occurring and the degree of fetal risk.

In a few severe cases, in which it is thought that the fetus will die before it is mature enough to survive delivery, intra-uterine transfusion may be performed. After ultrasonic localization of the placenta and fetus a needle is passed through the abdominal wall into the fetal peritoneal cavity, into which packed Rh negative red cells are injected. Absorption is surprisingly complete.

Alternatively circulating maternal rhesus antibodies can be removed by plasma electrophoresis, and this procedure may now replace intrauterine transfusion.

Iso-immunization to AB groups

If the fetus has an A or B blood group which is not possessed by the mother, haemolytic disease might be expected to occur. In fact it is rare, because A and B substances occur in all fetal tissues, so that most of the antibodies are absorbed by cells other than red blood cells. Although a few cases of O/A haemolytic disease occur these are very mild and seldom require exchange transfusion, but they may occur in first pregnancies. The Coombs' test is unreliable in these cases, but the mother's blood contains a rising titre of A haemolysins.

10

Obstetric operations

INDUCTION OF LABOUR

Labour may be started by induction before term, or after term in cases of postmaturity.

Indications

Induction should not be performed for the convenience of the doctor or the hospital, but if it is to be done a time should be chosen that is likely to lead to delivery when skilled staff are available. In about 20 per cent of pregnancies one of the following indications for induction will arise, for which reference to other chapters should be made.

1. Pre-eclampsia and eclampsia.
2. Essential hypertension.
3. Chronic nephritis.
4. Hydramnios.
5. Antepartum haemorrhage.
6. Disproportion.
7. Unstable lie.
8. Postmaturity.
9. Diabetes.
10. Haemolytic disease.
11. Anencephaly and other malformations.
12. Fetal death.

With modern methods induction in late pregnancy is nearly always successful, but it must be realized that failure leads to Caesarean section, and with amniotomy there is a small risk of cord prolapse or of infection. If there is any uncertainty about maturity induction may result in the birth of a premature infant. The indication and risk in each case must be carefully weighed; there is no place for routine induction nor for induction for the convenience of the attendants.

143

Failure is more likely if the presenting part is not engaged, if the cervix is long, firm and tightly closed, and before the 36th week. If a primigravida needs to be delivered before the 34th week Caesarean section is sometimes preferable to induction.

Methods of induction

The method which is now coming into general use is to insert a pessary in the vaginal vault which releases prostaglandin E_2 slowly. If uterine contractions do not follow the membranes may be ruptured by passing a small hook ('Amnihook') through the cervix, or with toothed forceps. Scrupulous aseptic technique is essential; anaesthesia is not usually required. A good deal of liquor should be let out, and a final examination made to exclude prolapse of the cord.

If progressive cervical dilatation does not follow at the normal rate (about 1 cm per hour) an intravenous syntocinon infusion is started.

Two units are added to 500 ml of dextrose solution and this is run at 40 drops per minute. The rate of the drip is regulated according to the uterine contractions, which must be carefully observed. Fetal death or uterine rupture can occur if the drip is not carefully supervised, and the method is only suitable for hospital practice. Automatic machines are available which regulate the infusion according to the rate of the contractions, but any ordinary drip can be used so long as the control is accurate. A tocograph and fetal scalp electrode are especially useful for monitoring these cases.

VERSION

External version

This is employed to correct a transverse lie, especially of a second twin (p. 111), or for breech presentation (see p. 97).

Internal version

In internal version the whole hand is passed into the uterus to grasp the feet. This is only possible after the cervix is fully dilated.

In the past many obstetric difficulties were overcome by turning the fetus and applying traction to the feet (podalic version). Today internal version is rarely employed except for a few cases of shoulder presentation (p. 100) or for delivery of a second twin.

DELIVERY WITH THE FORCEPS

History
The Chamberlen family were Huguenots who fled to England in 1569. The forceps were devised by one of them (probably Peter who died in 1631) and the invention was kept secret for about a century.

Description
There are innumerable types of forceps, but only three are in common use:

1. *Long curved forceps* (e.g., Neville's). There are two blades, each with its handle. The blades are inserted separ-

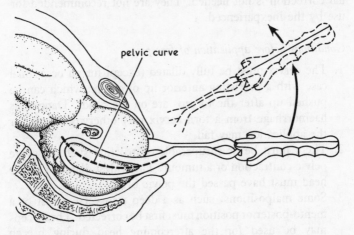

pelvic curve

Fig. 18 Forceps delivery.

ately and then the handles are locked together. Each blade has a cephalic curve (to fit the head) and a pelvic curve.

This type of forceps is used for delivery of the head from the pelvic cavity (mid-forceps delivery). Delivery of the head from above the pelvic brim (high forceps delivery) is dangerous and is not now performed.

The long curved forceps must always be applied correctly to the sides of the head. Because of the pelvic curve the forceps can only be applied in the anterior position — if the head is not in the antero-posterior diameter of the pelvis it must be rotated manually before applying the forceps. This instrument is not used for rotation.

2. *Short curved forceps* (e.g., Wrigley's). These light forceps may be used when the head is on the perineum (low forceps delivery).

3. *Kielland's forceps.* These are of different design. The pelvic curve is slight and the whole instrument is straighter. The lock allows the blades to slide on each other longitudinally, and (unlike other types) either blade can be inserted first. After correct application to the head the forceps can be used for rotation as well as traction, so that preliminary manual correction is not needed. They are not recommended for use by the inexperienced.

Conditions before application of forceps:

1. The cervix must be fully dilated (except for an occasional case with a persisting anterior lip of cervix, which can be pushed up after the forceps are on the head). Dangerous haemorrhage from a torn cervix may otherwise occur, or the application may fail.

2. There must be no insuperable obstruction such as severe pelvic contraction or a tumour. The widest diameter of the head must have passed the pelvic brim.

3. Some malpositions, such as a deep transverse arrest or a mento-posterior position must first be corrected. The forceps may be used for the aftercoming head during breech delivery.

It is also desirable that the bladder should be empty, the membranes should be ruptured, and the uterus should have sufficient tone to prevent postpartum haemorrhage.

Indications
1. Delay in the second stage:
   a. Inadequate uterine action or poor voluntary effort.
   b. Resistant perineum.
   c. Malposition of the head (after correction) such as posterior or lateral position of the occiput (p. 91), mentoposterior position (p. 93), brow presentation in the pelvic cavity (p. 94).
   d. Minor outlet disproportion (p. 105).
2. Maternal distress in the second stage
   No patient should be left for more than an hour in the second stage, and even earlier intervention is required if no progress is being made.
   Forceps may also be used to assist patients who are exhausted from a long first stage, and those with cardiac or pulmonary lesions or eclampsia.
3. Fetal distress in the second stage
   This may have no obvious cause, or may be due to prolapse of the cord or to placental insufficiency from pre-eclampsia, haemorrhage or postmaturity.

Maternal dangers
General anaesthesia is dangerous with an unprepared patient and inadequate facilities. The risk can often be avoided by using a pudendal block. Dangerous cervical, vaginal or perineal damage, sepsis, or postpartum haemorrhage are unlikely with ordinary care. Failure to deliver with the forceps, usually because of neglect to observe the conditions set out above, greatly increases all these dangers, and there may then be the hazard of subsequent Caesarean section or craniotomy.

Fetal dangers
Death may be due to intracranial haemorrhage (p. 169) and

skull fractures can occur. A common injury is facial palsy due to pressure on the VIIth nerve; complete recovery usually occurs.

Technique

The lithotomy position is usual, but if a general anaesthetic is used an experienced anaesthetist must be available and the table must be one that can be tilted quickly if the patient vomits. After applying antiseptic cream to the vulva, sterile towels are placed. If a difficult extraction is anticipated it is wise to empty the bladder with a catheter, but for a simple low forceps delivery this can be omitted. A vaginal examination is made to ensure that the conditions given above are satisfied, and to determine the position of the head accurately. If the sutures are obscured an ear must be felt. Episiotomy is usually needed.

Before applying ordinary forceps the head is rotated manually, if necessary, so as to bring the occiput to the anterior position. Because of the design of the lock of the forceps the left blade must always be inserted first. This blade is held vertically in the left hand and the fingers of the other hand are used to direct it between the head and the perineum. The handle is then swung down so that the blade passes up to the left side of the pelvis under the guidance of the internal fingers. If it is correctly placed it will not need to be held.

The right blade is now passed in a similar way, changing hands, and the handles are locked. If they will not lock easily the blades are not properly applied to the head. They must be removed and reapplied after the head has been correctly rotated.

Traction must be intermittent, and with the pains if they are frequent enough. The pull is obliquely towards the floor at first. As the head descends the handles tend to rise, and the direction of traction is gradually altered so that when the head reaches the vulval orifice the pull is towards the ceiling (Fig. 18). The handles can be removed for crowning, or left in place to control the head.

With *Kielland's forceps* the instrument should first be articulated outside the pelvis and held so that the slight pelvic curve is directed towards the occiput to ensure that the forceps are correctly orientated. If the head does not need rotation the blades are applied as already described, but if the head is lying transversely or obliquely the *anterior* blade is selected and inserted first, by passing it into the sacral hollow behind the head and then 'wandering' it around the head until it lies over the anterior ear. The posterior blade is then applied. The head can be rotated with the forceps, and this is easiest if the head is lifted up a little at the same time.

Undue force should not be used for either traction or rotation during foreceps delivery.

VACUUM EXTRACTOR (VENTOUSE)

This consists of a metal suction cup (supplied in three sizes) which is applied to the fetal scalp. The cup is connected to a vacuum pump by a rubber tube, and there is a chain by means of which traction can be applied to the cup. When a negative pressure (maximum 0.8 kg/cm^2) is produced in the cup the scalp is drawn into it forming a 'chignon', and a firm hold is obtained. The cup should be applied over the occiput. Anaesthesia is not required, and the smaller cups can be applied before the cervix is fully dilated. If the occiput is situated posteriorly it will often rotate during traction. The cap should not be left in place for more than 30 minutes for fear of cephalhaematoma or scalp necrosis.

The ventouse can be used instead of forceps, but in cases of fetal distress forceps delivery may be quicker and therefore preferable. It may also be used in cases of prolonged first stage due to abnormal uterine action when the cervix is more than half dilated, but it should never be used in cases of disproportion.

PUDENDAL BLOCK

It is convenient to mention this here. Lignocaine 1 per cent is used, up to a total of 40 ml. The index finger is placed in the vagina and the ischial spine can then be felt on the side wall of the pelvis. A 10 cm needle is inserted through the vaginal wall to reach a point below and beyond the ischial spine, where 10 ml of solution is injected. The posterior part of the labium majus, which is separately innervated, is also infiltrated with another 5 ml of solution. The technique is repeated on the opposite side.

EPIDURAL ANALGESIA

This may also be mentioned here. It is a most effective method of relieving pain, suitable for both normal labour and operative vaginal delivery. It is usually started during the first stage. A needle is inserted into the epidural space by the lumbar route. (The space can also be approached through the sacral hiatus, but such *caudal analgesia* is now seldom employed). Bupivicaine 0.25 per cent is injected. A polythene catheter is passed through the needle and left in place so that the injection can be 'topped up' as necessary.

Some experience is required in placing the needle and the method is usually in the hands of anaesthetists rather than obstetricians, but whoever is responsible must be able to deal with unexpected complications such as hypotension or temporary respiratory paralysis if the injection inadvertently enters the theca. Uterine tone is normal, or even raised, but voluntary expulsive effort is often impaired, so that low forceps or vacuum extraction is often required.

CAESAREAN SECTION

History
Julius Caesar was not delivered in this way. The name may derive from a Roman law which directed that the child should be removed from any woman who died in childbirth. Various attempts, mostly fatal from haemorrhage or sepsis, were made

to perform the operation in the 17th and 18th centuries, but it was not until 1882 that Sänger perfected the classical (upper segment) operation. During labour this was still hazardous from infection until Frank introduced the lower segment operation in 1906.

Indications

These are usually relative and seldom absolute. Factors are often combined, e.g., section might be chosen for breech delivery with an android pelvis, but not for either of these alone. The risk of section is about ten times that of vaginal delivery, but this maternal risk is acceptable for some fetal indications (e.g., breech delivery) if the mother has little hope of a later successful pregnancy because of age, infertility or her obstetric history, wheras in a young normal patient vaginal delivery would be chosen. It is easy to perform a section — the decision when to do it requires experience. Section is indicated in *some* instances of the following cases. The student will find it instructive to work out the indication in each case.

Maternal and fetal indications

1. Disproportion.
2. Pelvic tumours.
3. Malpresentations; breech, brow, shoulder.
4. Abnormal uterine action.
5. Antepartum haemorrhage.
6. Pre-eclampsia, eclampsia and essential hypertension.

Fetal indications

7. Fetal distress in the first stage of labour, due to prolonged labour, prolapsed cord, placental insufficiency, or sometimes with no explanation.
8. Placental insufficiency; when the fetus is not growing or placental function tests are adverse section is sometimes preferable to induction of labour.
9. Diabetes.

Maternal indications

10. After some operations for prolapse or fistula.
11. Previous Caesarean section. If the section was for a persisting indication (e.g., disproportion) another section is required, but if it was for a non-recurrent indication (e.g., placenta praevia), in spite of a small risk of scar rupture, vaginal delivery in hospital is safer than repeated section.

Preparation

Caesarean section is often an emergency operation during labour, but elective operations are best performed a week before term.

Purges and enemas are unnecessary and vaginal 'purification' is dangerous. A catheter is passed in the theatre. Drugs such as morphine which would depress the fetal respiratory centre are not used. The risk of acid regurgitation is reduced by giving 2 g of magnesium trisilicate in a little water. All preparations must be completed before the anaesthetic is begun so that the child can be delivered expeditiously.

Blood is taken beforehand for cross-matching, and in cases of placenta praevia blood must be immediately available.

Anaesthesia

Many methods are used by experts. For an elective case a small dose of thiopentone may be followed by nitrous oxide and oxygen, and relaxants (with a cuffed tracheal tube) are often given. Alternatively lumbar extradural anaesthesia is often chosen.

Lower segment operation

This is now the standard procedure. To prevent compression of the inferior vena cava and obstruction to the venous return it is best to have the patient tilted laterally by using a 15° wedge until the baby is delivered. The abdomen is opened through a midline or transverse subumbilical incision and a wide Doyen retractor is inserted at the lower end. Packing the abdomen with gauze has no advantage. The peritoneum just above the bladder is incised transversely, and slight downward displacement of the bladder exposes the lower segment, which is also incised transversely. The fetal head is lifted out with the hand or with Wrigley's forceps, and the shoulders are eased out. If the breech presents it is delivered by groin traction.

As soon as the mouth is free it is sucked out (a sterile attachment to the suction machine should be available). The child is held at the same level as the placenta in the uterus with its head downwards while the cord is divided, and then passed to an assistant. While the placenta is being delivered by cord traction the anaesthetist gives an intravenous injection of ergometrine 0.5 mg.

The uterine muscle is repaired with two layers of Dexon or chromic catgut, avoiding the endometrium. The uterovesical peritoneum is sutured with fine catgut. After sucking or mopping out any blood and liquor the abdomen is closed in the usual way.

Classical section

This is no longer classical, and should simply be called the upper segment operation. It is obsolete except when the lower segment is inaccessible (e.g., from fibroids), and even for placenta praevia the lower incision is preferable.

A paramedian incision with one-third above the umbilicus is made. The uterus is incised in the midline and the fetus is extracted feet first.

The lower incision is better (even if there is not a well-formed lower segment before labour) because:

1. There is less risk of general peritonitis in infected cases.
2. The incision bleeds less and suturing is easier. It heals better as it is more quiescent in the puerperium. Subsequent rupture during pregnancy is rare, and rupture during labour is less dangerous than with an upper segment scar.

Sterilization

This may be performed at the time of Caesarean section but the operation should never be done just to permit this.

Postoperative care

This is the same as that after any laparotomy.

Maternal dangers

The immediate risks are those of any abdominal operation but four are especially important:

1. Those of anaesthesia in an unprepared patient.
2. Haemorrhage, especially in cases of antepartum haemorrhage.
3. Sepsis, in cases of prolonged labour.
4. Pulmonary embolism (p. 133).

Late complications include rupture of the scar in a subsequent pregnancy or labour.

Fetal dangers

The fetal mortality after section is relatively high, but in most cases this is because of the indication for the operation (e.g., fetal distress) or prematurity, rather than due to the operation itself.

SYMPHYSIOTOMY

The symphysis pubis can be divided through a small suprapubic incision to allow the pelvic ring to expand slightly. This operation is seldom performed in Britain, but has its advocates in countries where a Caesarean scar may mean disaster in a subsequent unsupervised labour.

DESTRUCTIVE OPERATIONS

These are now seldom required in Britain.

Craniotomy
This is performed:

1. If the fetus is dead and labour is obstructed. (Caesarean Section is often safer, especially of the head is high.)
2. For hydrocephaly (p. 100).

The perforator is an instrument with triangular blades which come together to form a point. After insertion of the point into the skull the blades are separated widely. If the head does not collapse sufficiently after making a cruciate opening in the skull the cranioclast is used. This is a heavy (and dangerous) crushing instrument.

Decapitation
Decapitation is rarely required for a neglected shoulder presentation with a dead fetus (p. 100) or for locked twins (p. 111).

Cleidotomy
Division of the clavicles may allow delivery of impacted shoulders after fetal death.

Embryotomy
Various other destructive operations are rarely performed for double monsters, fetal ascites or fetal tumours obstructing delivery.

AMNIOCENTESIS

A sample of liquor amnii can be obtained by inserting a needle through the anterior abdominal wall into the uterine cavity. There is a small risk of causing placental bleeding, of introducing fetal red cells into the maternal circulation, or of injuring the fetus. It is an advantage if the placental site and fetal portion are determined by ultrasound, so that the needle can be directed to avoid them.

Indications

1. In early pregnancy amniotic cells may be grown in tissue culture to detect chromosomal abnormalities, or to determine fetal sex in cases of sex-linked inheritable disease. The incidence of Down's syndrome (trisomy 21) increases with maternal age, reaching 2 per cent in mothers older than 40. In these patients and those who already have a mongol child amniocentesis may be considered.

2. If the fetus has an open neural tube defect alpha-fetoprotein escapes into the liquor in increased amounts. The discovery of a high concentration in liquor (or in maternal serum) calls for an ultrasonic examination to exclude anencephaly and gross spina bifida.

3. For bilirubin estimation in haemolytic disease. (See p. 141).

4. A test for the maturity of the fetal lung is to estimate the lecithin content of the liquor, usually expressed as a ratio against the sphingomyelin content. The L:S ratio is an index of the surfactant activity of the fetal lung; with a ratio above 2 respiratory distress syndrome is unlikely to occur (p. 162).

OXYTOCIC DRUGS

For convenience a note about these is included here.

Ergot

Ergot is a crude extract of a fungus that grows on rye. There are several active substances but the most important for obstetrics is *ergometrine*. The dose of 0.5 mg can be given orally, intramuscularly or intravenously, and the respective times before it acts are about 7 minutes, 4 minutes and $\frac{1}{2}$ minute. The time can be shortened after intramuscular injection by adding hyalase. It causes strong and persisting uterine spasm, and should never be used before the third stage of labour for fear of uterine rupture or fetal death. It can safely be used in cases of abortion.

Posterior pituitary extract

Oxytocin (Pitocin) is secreted by the posterior lobe of the pituitary gland, and causes strong uterine contractions in late pregnancy. It has less effect in early pregnancy, and it has little or no effect on the blood pressure, intestine or kidney. Oxytocin is an amino-acid complex which is destroyed in the alimentary tract, and is therefore given by intravenous infusion. This also allows the dose to be accurately controlled. The standard preparation contains 10 units per ml. In small doses it accentuates rhythmical contractions, but large doses can rupture the uterus or kill the fetus. It is used for induction of labour, augmentation of labour or post-partum haemorrhage.

Syntocinon

This is a synthetic preparation which corresponds in action and dosage to oxytocin and now used in place of it.

Syntometrine

Syntometrine contains 5 units of Syntocinon and 0.5 mg of ergometrine per ml. It is given as an intramuscular injection. The Syntocinon acts after about 2½ minutes, and the subsequent action of the ergometrine maintains the uterine contraction.

Prostaglandins

These are a group of long-chain unsaturated fatty acids, originally found in semen but now known to occur in many tissues. Prostaglandin E_2 causes strong uterine contractions when given by intravenous drip, and has been used to induce labour or abortion. Prostaglandins are also absorbed from the vagina. Vaginal pessaries which release PGE_2 slowly are convenient for induction of labour. They are available in forms containing 2, 4 or 10 mg of PGE_2.

11

Care of the newborn child

ASPHYXIA NEONATORUM

Immediately after delivery the establishment of respiration takes precedence over all else. In utero the fetus makes periodic respiratory movements which are sufficient to draw amniotic fluid into the bronchial tree. Immediately after delivery there is mild hypoxia, with a fall in Po_2 and a rise in Pco_2. The respiratory centre of the newborn infant responds to the increased CO_2 concentration, and the response is fortified by a variety of peripheral stimuli, including cold and contact of a catheter on the pharynx. If the infant becomes more severely hypoxic the respiratory centre does not respond to these stimuli ('primary apnoea') but after a time irregular gasping respiration occurs, partly due to impulses arising from the carotid and aortic chemoreceptors during oxygen lack. Finally, if the hypoxia is still not relieved the respiratory centre is paralysed and will not respond at all ('secondary apnoea').

When respiration is established air is drawn into the alveoli, which expand successively. To expand the lungs not only must their elastic recoil be overcome, but also the tendency of the alveolar walls to cohere. In late pregnancy alveolar cells secrete *surfactant*, a lipo-protein of which lecithin is a main component. This reduces surface tension and allows easier expansion.

As the lungs expand the pulmonary vessels open up, and the ductus arteriosus and the umbilical vessels contract. The ductus and the cord vessels have a natural tendency to contract, and it is believed that high fetal levels of prostaglandins keep them patent until after delivery. As the placental circulation ceases the left arterial pressure rises and the foramen ovale closes.

The infant's respiratory effort is chiefly diaphragmatic, and if the airway is obstructed the sternum will be indrawn with each breath. A negative pressure of 20 cm of water is required for pulmonary expansion.

Aetiology
Failure to breathe soon after birth may be due to:

1. Obstruction to the airway by mucus or meconium.
2. Damage to the respiratory centre by hypoxia before delivery, e.g., from a prolapsed cord, a placental lesion or long labour.
3. Depression of the respiratory centre by drugs such as morphine or pethidine given to the mother within two hours of delivery. Their effect can be counteracted by giving an injection of naloxone hydrochloride 0.01 mg/kg to the infant after birth.
4. Intracranial haemorrhage (p. 169).

Clinical events
Before a breath is taken the infant is cyanosed, but unless the hypoxia is prolonged the pulse rate is more than 100 per minute and the muscular tone is good. If hypoxia is prolonged, either before or after delivery, the circulation fails, the pulse rate is slow, and the blood flow in the skin is reduced so that the infant looks pale. Muscular tone is lost and there is no response to stimuli.

A mark of 0, 1 or 2 may be given for each of these five features: respiratory effort, pulse rate, colour, muscular tone and response to stimuli, and the total gives the 'Apgar score', ranging from 0 to 10.

Treatment

It can be lifesaving to have a doctor experienced in neonatal resuscitation present at the delivery of any infant likely to need this, e.g., pre-term infants, cases of fetal distress, Caesarean section, breech or twin delivery.

Immediately after delivery the pharynx and nasal passages are cleared with a soft plastic catheter. Appropriate equipment for further treatment must always be ready. If respiration does not start after clearing the pharynx the baby is placed head downwards on an inclined plane and a laryngoscope is passed. A fine endotracheal tube is inserted and the trachea is cleared by suction. The tube is attached to a water manometer and a suitable supply of oxygen. The lungs are intermittently inflated (for 2 seconds 12 times per minute) at a pressure of 25 cm of water. When spontaneous respiratory efforts begin oxygen is given with a small face mask. If the heart stops external cardiac massage may be tried.

There is no satisfactory evidence that other forms of artificial respiration, or such drugs as nikethamide, lobeline, vanillic ethylamide or adrenaline do good.

Facilities for chemical control should be available, but acidosis is more often overcome by establishment of respiration than by intravenous (umbilical) administration of alkali and glucose.

Outside hospital, without equipment in an emergency, mouth-to-mouth respiration or oral inflation through a fine intratracheal tube are justifiable.

Continuing respiratory distress

Respiratory distress may continue or may first appear some hours after birth. Immediate transfer to a neonatal special care unit is essential. The following conditions require consideration:

Atelectasis

Part or all of the alveoli may be collapsed and airless. This may be a primary condition in small premature infants. It may occur by secondary absorption of gas beyond bronchioles obstructed by meconium, hyaline membrane or inflammation. Periodic apnoeic phases occur.

Hyaline membrane disease (Respiratory distress syndrome)

In premature infants, including infants of diabetic mothers, a few hours after birth a fibrinous exudate may form in the smaller bronchioles and alveoli. The cause is uncertain. There is a relative deficiency of surfactant in the premature infant, and this may be increased by hypoxia. With the hypoxia and atelectasis the pulmonary circulation closes down and much of the blood is shunted through the foramen ovale and ductus arteriosus.

Severe respiratory distress occurs, with cyanosis and indrawing of the ribs and sternum. A radiograph shows fine mottling due to patchy atelectasis. The mortality is high, but those who survive to the third day may recover completely.

If there is doubt about the maturity of the fetal lung before delivery the lecithin content of the liquor may be estimated as an indication of the surfactant level. It is claimed that intramuscular injection of dexamethasone (4 mg 6 hourly) to the mother for 2 days before delivery will improve maturation of the fetal lung.

Air accident

Mediastinal emphysema or a pneumothorax may occur. The radiological appearances are obvious, and needling may relieve distress due to pneumothorax.

Infective bronchopneumonia

This may follow long labour.

Pulmonary haemorrhage

Pulmonary haemorrhage can occur into the alveoli.

In the management of all these conditions the administration of oxygen and naso-gastric feeding will be required, sometimes with the correction of respiratory acidosis by intravenous injection of sodium bicarbonate, and the use of antibiotics in cases of infection.

OTHER IMMEDIATE CARE

Eyes and mouth

The eyes and mouth are *not* mopped with wool or gauze; this might introduce infection and certainly would not remove it. Credè's method of instillation of a drop of silver nitrate solution (1 per cent) into each eye to prevent gonococcal infection is not now practised in Britain, but may still be justified in some places where the infants are not well supervised. Also see p. 174.

Prevention of hypothermia

In the newborn infant the heat-regulating mechanism is ineffective and it is essential to prevent undue heat loss, either by wrapping the baby in a warm towel and blanket, or in hospital by the use of a radiant heat device. Heat regulation is partly effected by metabolism of brown fat, which is deficient in small infants.

Bathing

The newborn baby is covered with *vernix caseosa*, a cheesy substance consisting of sebaceous secretion with epithelial cells. This should be left alone and the traditional birthday bath should be abandoned. Until the cord has separated cleaning is restricted to the napkin area.

Care of the cord

The cord stump dries and usually separates by granulation in seven days. It is important to prevent umbilical infection and many techniques are in use. One is to tie the cord at about 3 cm with sterile thick linen thread. A good alternative is to use a sterile disposable plastic clip, which is applied close to the skin and crushes the cord; it can be removed after 48 hours. The stump is left exposed but painted daily with chlor-hexidine, 1 per cent in spirit. Chlorhexidine powder may also be applied.

Breast engorgement

The breast may show engorgement in both male and female infants from transfer of maternal oestrogens. No treatment is required.

Examination

Soon after birth the baby is carefully and systematically examined for any congenital abnormality. The passage of urine and meconium is observed. If meconium is not passed in the first day the rectum is examined. A test for congenital dislocation of the hip joint is made, and on the 7th day a Guthrie test for phenylketonuria. A second complete examination should be made on leaving hospital or on the 10th day.

Identification

In hospital every baby should have an identification tape sewn around the wrist.

Prevention of infection

Infants are susceptible to infection. They are best kept separately, each with its mother ('rooming in'), although noisy babies may have to be removed to a nursery. Before any attention the mother or nurse must wash her hands carefully. Any infected baby is isolated.

BREAST FEEDING

A textbook of paediatrics must be consulted for further details. Breast feeding should be encouraged because with it infection is less likely, the composition of the milk is more suitable than that provided by cows, and there are psychological advantages ('bonding') in the close contact of mother and baby. A healthy baby is first put to the breast for a short time immediately after delivery. The baby's cot is kept beside the mother's bed for the first few weeks, and even in hospital 'on demand' feeding is preferable to a fixed routine. The early feeds may be short and at frequent and irregular intervals, but it is usually found that a regular rhythm of 4-hourly feeds with about 10 minutes at each breast becomes established. For the first 2 days yellow colostrum is secreted (p. 41) which has a high content of protein antibodies.

After feeding on each side the baby is held up to get rid of wind. Before and after feeds the nipples are cleaned with a swab dipped in boiled water.

The best stimulus to lactation is regular suckling. After the 7th day the average requirements is 150 ml of milk per kg of baby per day. Thirty ml of milk should give 20 calories (4200 J).

Contraindications to breast feeding are few. Rare maternal contraindications are severe cardiac disease, tuberculosis with positive sputum, and puerperal psychosis.

A baby suffering from intracranial injury, respiratory distress or infection may be unable to feed and require tube feeding for a time. Although breast milk is always desirable for them, very small premature infants may also fail to feed at the breast. Retracted nipples, cleft lip or cleft palate may prevent feeding. For engorgement of the breast see p. 130, cracked nipple, p. 131, and mastitis p. 131. If the baby is to be immediately adopted breast feeding is not attempted.

ARTIFICIAL FEEDING

Cow's milk always contains a wide variety of bacteria and it must always be sterilized for infant feeding. Cow's milk differs in composition from human milk:

	Protein %	Fat %	Lactose %
Human milk	1.25	3.5	7
Cow's milk	3.5	3.5	4.5

The protein is almost all caseinogen and lactalbumin. Cow's milk contains a much larger proportion of the less digestible caseinogen. The fat globules in cow's milk are larger.

Dried milk or evaporated milk preparations are now almost universally used. The drying process partly breaks down the protein, but also destroys vitamins, which must be added. Full-cream preparations have the same fat content as raw milk. Half-cream preparations are made from milk which has been skimmed to remove fat and to which sugar has been added. Low solute preparations which are more sophisticated and more closely resemble breast milk in composition and osmolar qualities are now preferred to half-cream preparations. Paediatric textbooks contain exhaustive (and exhausting) lists of various artificial feeds.

For simplicity:
Feeding is begun with a low solute preparation, made up with water according to the maker's instructions. Starting with 30 ml/Kg/day, the amount is gradually increased so that the baby is getting 150/Kg/day after about a week. The feeds may be given 3-hourly at first, but later 4-hourly. A change to a full-cream preparation may subsequently be made.

In hospitals prepacked feeds which only require the attachment of a teat to the bottle may be available.

SMALL INFANTS

It was formerly the practice to designate any baby weighing less than 2500 g at birth as 'premature', whatever the duration of the pregnancy, because records of weight were more likely to be accurate than those of duration. It is now usual to describe these as babies of 'low birth weight'. Two classes are included; babies born before term but of normal weight for the length of gestation, and growth-retarded babies that are 'small-for-dates'. (Some babies fall into both categories). Tables are available that give the expected range of weights for each week of pregnancy. Growth-retarded fetuses have a high risk of intra-uterine or perinatal death. Babies born before 28 weeks, with an expected weight of less than 1100 g are regarded as non-viable, although a few of them survive. The mortality among babies of low birth weight is high from intracranial haemorrhage, pulmonary complications, infection and feeding difficulties. Kernicterus (p. 140) and haemorrhagic disease (p. 172) may also occur. With babies of between 1100 and 1600 g the mortality is as high as 40 per cent, but with those over 2000 g it is only 4 per cent.

Aetiology and prevention

The incidence of low birth weight is about 7 per cent. No cause is found in about a third of the cases, and about half the remainder follow induction of labour. Common causes of the fetus being small-for-dates are pre-eclampsia and hypertension, multiple pregnancy and antepartum haemorrhage. Fetal abnormalities account for a smaller number of cases. The incidence of low birth weight is higher in poorer families and with mothers who smoke heavily.

Improvement is only possible if these causes can be prevented or treated, which is hardly the case at present. If premature labour is a possibility delivery should be in hospital.

Management

Special medical and nursing experience contributes greatly to success. Paediatric textbooks should be consulted, but immediate treatment includes:

1. *Management of respiratory difficulties.* See pp. 159 et seq.
2. *Maintenance of body temperature.* Babies weighing less than 2 kg should be transferred to a special unit. Particular care must be taken not to expose small babies during resuscitation. Small babies are nursed in incubators, where they can be left undisturbed in a moist warm atmosphere (33°C or more) and unclothed to allow free respiration and movement. Larger babies may be in cots, but the room should be kept at 27°C.

3. *Prevention of infection*. Measures include isolation, exclusion of visitors except the parents, careful hand washing, and a separate gown for each cot. If there are pulmonary complications prophylactic antibiotics may be given.

4. *Feeding*. Small premature babies with poor swallowing reflexes can die from aspiration of regurgitated milk. They should not be fed orally until they show sucking movements. A fine polythene tube is passed through a nostril into the stomach. Any gastric fluid is aspirated and feeding can then be begun through the tube. Slightly larger babies who can swallow but not suck effectively are fed with a premature baby bottle, or from a spoon.

It may take over a fortnight to reach a daily intake of 150 ml of feed per kg weight per day, and the premature baby subsequently needs more than this, but there should be no hurry. Two-hourly feeds of diluted expressed breast milk are given at first, and slowly increased to full strength at longer intervals. If breast milk is not available a start may be made with a low solute preparation. Vitamins C and D should soon be added.

5. *Hypoglycaemia*. Small babies, and those with respiratory distress syndrome, may have low glycogen reserves and develop hypoglycaemia. There is twitching, convulsions, apathy and refusal to feed, and sometimes apnoea. The diagnosis is confirmed by Dextrostix tests on blood from a heel stab. Administration of glucose solution through a naso-gastric tube is usually adequate treatment.

Large babies of diabetic mothers may have hyperplasia of the pancreatic islets and hypoglycaemia because of high blood insulin levels. Early milk feeding may be all that is necessary, but in a few casses small doses of hydrocortisone are required.

6. *Hypocalcaemia*. Small newborn infants may develop twitching and tetany from hypocalcaemia, and the same condition may occur at about the 7th day in infants fed on high-solute artificial feeds. Calcium gluconate may be

added to the feeds, or in severe cases given cautiously intravenously.

7. *Kernicterus.* Premature babies may not be able to conjugate
bilirubin effectively, so that severe jaundice occurs with a
risk of kernicterus (p. 140). If the serum bilirubin exceeds
340 mmol/1 exchange transfusion may be required.

BIRTH INJURIES

Cephalhaematoma

A subperiosteal haematoma may occur over a parietal bone.
It is limited by the attachment of the periosteum to the edges
of the bone. Although absorption is slow and the haematoma
may ossify no treatment is required.

Fractures of the skull

These may follow forceps delivery through a contracted pelvis. They may be associated with intracranial haemorrhage.
Fractures which remain depressed, or those associated with
symptoms, should be elevated surgically and any haematoma
evacuated.

Intracranial haemorrhage

1. *Traumatic haemorrhage.* Blood vessels may be torn because
of excessive moulding of the head, particularly in cases of
disproportion, or of forceps or breech delivery, but the
accident can occur with normal labour, especially if it is
rapid. If the cerebral vault is displaced upwards by moulding the falx cerebri is under tension. This, or more commonly the tentorium cerebelli to which it is attached, gives
way, tearing adjacent vessels.
   Bleeding may occur in various sites:
      Extradural haemorrhage is uncommon except when a
   large sinus is torn, and then there is usually also subarachnoid haemorrhage.
      Subdural haemorrhage is also uncommon. A small vein

is torn between the dura and the arachnoid, and a localized haematoma slowly forms.

Subarachnoid haemorrhage is the common form of fatal intracranial haemorrhage. If the lateral sinus or the great cerebral vein of Galen is torn the bleeding is subtentorial. Occasionally a tear of the superior longitudinal sinus causes supratentorial bleeding.

2. *Anoxic haemorrhage.* Haemorrhage also occurs in cases of anoxia, especially in premature infants. A congested choroid plexus bleeds into the lateral ventricle, or petechial haemorrhages occur widely in the brain substance.

Clinical events

Major haemorrhages are fatal, minor haemorrhage is undiagnosed. Those of intermediate degree cause difficulty in establishment of respiration, often with pallor and a slow heart rate, and cyanotic attacks. There may be convulsions, twitching, strabismus and failure to suck. The infant may be restless with a persistent high-pitched cry, or drowsy. The fontanelle may be tense, and there may be rigidity of the neck. Recovery may be rapid and complete, or there may be persisting signs of cerebral damage, probably chiefly due to anoxia.

In cases of subdural haematoma signs appear slowly over some weeks, with failure to thrive, fits and other neurological signs. Needling the brain through the fontanelle may prove the diganosis.

Treatment. Except in cases of subdural haematoma or fracture of the skull bones surgical treatment is not recommended. The infant is disturbed as little as possible. If there are cyanotic attacks oxygen is given. Feeding is postponed for a time, and may have to be by tube. Nursing in an incubator is often convenient. Lumbar puncture is no help, but intracranial pressure can be reduced by the rectal instillation of 50 ml of 10 per cent saline. If the baby is restless intramuscular injections of paraldehyde 0.15 ml/kg may be given.

Nerve injuries

Facial palsy. See p. 148.

Brachial plexus injuries are uncommon but may result from forcible lateral flexion of the head during delivery. The commonest type is Erb's palsy, in which the 5th and 6th cervical nerves are damaged. Some of the shoulder muscles and the flexors of the elbow are paralysed, so that the arm lies internally rotated at the side of the trunk. Splinting is arranged to prevent stretching of the paralysed muscles, and a fair degree of recovery can be hoped for.

Fractures of the humerus, clavicle or femur

These are rare. With a fractured humerus the arm is strapped to the side, and with a fractured femur to the trunk in full flexion. Union is rapid and if alignment is bad it soon improves.

Visceral injuries

Hepatic injury is difficult to diagnose unless a haematoma is felt, when surgical treatment may be attempted. Adrenal haemorrhage may occur, with severe shock.

SOME OTHER ABNORMALITIES NEEDING EARLY RECOGNITION

The management of most of the following abnormalities will be the responsibility of the paediatrician and *a complete description is not attempted here*, but early suspicion of their presence is important.

Vomiting

Overfeeding or *failure to bring up wind* are simple explanations of most cases, but *obstructive vomiting* needs recognition.

If there is difficulty in swallowing, choking or unusual regurgitation, especially after hydramnios, an oesophageal catheter is passed. If this does not easily enter the stomach immediate investigation for oesophageal atresia or tracheo-oesophageal fistula is required.

Obstruction may be due to duodenal or ileal atresia, mal-rotation of the gut or meconium ileus. The last is due to lack of pancreatic enzymes so that undigested meconium forms a putty-like mass. With obstruction there is persistent vomiting, usually bile stained, abdominal distension, visible peristalsis and failure to pass meconium. An X-ray will show dilatation of part of the gut with fluid levels. Surgical exploration is urgently required.

An imperforate anus should be discovered at the first examination.

With a diaphragmatic hernia a lot of the abdominal contents may pass into the chest, and there is both vomiting and cyanosis. Respiratory sounds are absent from one side, and may be replaced by bowel sounds. An X-ray is conclusive.

Symptoms of pyloric stenosis or pylorospasm seldom appear before the second week.

Vomiting may occur with gastro-enteritis or other infections.

Diarrhoea

In the young infant this may be due to:

1. Feeding difficulties — feeds which are increased too fast or which contain too much fat or sugar.
2. Infectious enteritis.
3. Parenteral infections such as pyelonephritis.

Haemorrhage

Prothrombin deficiency (haemorrhagic disease). From the 2nd to the 7th day the infant's blood prothrombin level is low, especially in premature infants. Haemorrhage may occur from the stomach (haematemesis) or bowel (melaena), or less commonly in the lungs, brain, skin or elsewhere. An intramuscular injection of phytomenadione (vitamin K_1) 1 mg will alow the liver to form prothrombin until the vitamin is absorbed in the usual way from the bowel.

(Vomiting of blood may occur because the infant has swallowed it from a cracked nipple.)

Umbilical haemorrhage can occur if the ligature is not properly applied, or as a secondary haemorrhage from infection.

Thrombocytopenic purpura may be a transient event in the newborn if the mother has this disease.

Uterine bleeding can occur from withdrawal of the effect of the maternal oestrogens.

Jaundice

Physiological jaundice. At birth the infant at term has a high red cell count (more than six million RBC per mm³) and haemoglobin concentration (16 g per 100 ml). After birth some of the excess red cells are haemolysed. The liver, especially of the premature infant, may not be able to conjugate all the bilirubin which is released, so that jaundice occurs, starting on about the second day and persisting for a week. The colour is seldom deep, the liver is not enlarged, and the stools are normal.

Natural recovery is to be expected, but cases that do not quickly improve may be helped by whole body exposure to ultraviolet light, taking care to cover the eyes. In premature infants the bilirubin level may rise dangerously (340 mmol/l) so that there is a risk of kernicterus and exchange transfusion is sometimes required (p. 141).

Infective jaundice. Umbilical sepsis may spread to the liver, or virus hepatitis may occur. Syphilis and toxoplasmosis can affect the liver.

Congenital atresia of the bile ducts causes deep jaundice with pale stools and hepatic enlargement. Surgery may be attempted.

Haemolytic disease. See p. 138.

Other rare causes of jaundice in the newborn include congenital spherocytic anaemia, cretinism, glucose-6-phosphate dehydrogenase deficiency and galactosaemia.

Anaemia

Anaemia is rare as a result of haemolytic disease or haemorrhage (from a slipped cord ligature, division of placental vessels at Caesarean section, or after circumcision).

Infection

The newborn infant has a poor resistance to bacterial infection. This is particularly true of small premature infants, and with modern intensive care more such infants survive to be at risk. Fulminant multisystemic invasion may occur from infection during labour, or later less acute infection may come from human contacts. Septicaemia or meningitis may occur. Bacterial infection may be with *E. coli, Staph. aureus* or streptococci, especially of group B. Viral infections also occur Symptoms are often misleading or absent, and fever may be slight. Any infection may cause refusal to feed, or vomiting and diarrhoea, and as a result rapid dehydration may occur. Maintenance of fluid and electrolyte balance may require great skill. There should be no hesitation in securing a blood culture or performing a lumbar puncture, and the urine must be carefully examined in every case. It is not possible to wait for the results of bacterial investigation if the baby is very ill. Treatment is begun with a wide spectrum antibiotic (e.g., cloxacillin 50 mg per kg three times daily) and revised later. All infected infants must be isolated.

Conjunctivitis (ophthalmia neonatorum). Before the introduction of antibiotics there was a serious risk of blindness with gonococcal infection and Credè's prophylaxis by insertion of silver nitrate drops was used. Today infection is far more often due to staphylococci, diphtheroids or other organisms. While bacterial swabs are being examined penicillin eye drops are instilled every 15 minutes for the first 6 hours, and then 3-hourly. Local treatment is given according to the result. Eye drops are available containing sulphacetamide, penicillin or chloramphenicol, and ointment containing chlortetracycline.

Skin infection. Staphylococci often cause small pustules. Pemphigus is now rare. This used to occur in epidemics and was due to particular strains of staphylococci which caused a generalized eruption of large vesicles containing thin pus. Oral antibiotics are given and the skin is painted with a mixture of brilliant green and crystal violet ($\frac{1}{2}$ per cent of each) in spirit.

Umbilical infection. Prevention (p. 163) is very important, as infection may spread along the umbilical vein to the liver.

Thrush. Oral infection with *Candida albicans* (monilia) may occur if the mother has vaginitis. White plaques occur from which the organism is easily cultured. The mouth is painted with nystatin 100 000 units per ml, or with gentian violet 1 per cent.

Pneumonia may follow long labor when organisms are aspirated before or during delivery, or may be due to descending infection from the upper respiratory tract, or to haematogenous spread. Coughing does not occur. Rapid respiration and cyanosis may be seen, but physical signs are often few unless an X-ray is taken. Infection with group B streptococci from the maternal genital tract may be especially dangerous.

Gastroenteritis. This is extremely dangerous and immediate expert treatment is essential.

Pyelonephritis may cause an obscure illness at the end of the first week, often with vomitting and diarrhoea but not urinary symptoms. An examination of the urine for pus cells should never be omitted.

Osteomyelitis may give no local signs at first except that the infant keeps the limb still.

Syphilis. See p. 84.

Convulsions or repetitive jerky movements may result from:

1. Cerebral trauma.
2. Infections (e.g., meningitis).
3. Hypoglycaemia, especially in babies of low birth weight or diabetic mothers.
4. Hypocalcaemia (>1.8 mmol/l plasma) especially in artificially fed infants.

12

Vital statistics

Reliable statistics are only available in countries with advanced medical and social services. In what follows any figures only relate to Britain.

Maternal mortality
The *maternal mortality rate* is defined as the number of deaths ascribed to pregnancy and childbearing per thousand live and stillbirths. Deaths from abortion should be included although they are often tabulated separately. The present rate is about 0.12 per thousand of which abortion accounts for 0.01 per thousand.

According to the Confidential Reports of the Ministry of Health in England and Wales (1972–75) the chief causes of maternal death are:

Obstetric causes	Per cent of deaths
Hypertensive disease	12
Antepartum haemorrhage	2
Postpartum haemorrhage	3
Puerperal infection (other than postabortal)	6
Pulmonary embolism	10
Amniotic fluid embolism	4
Abortion (including legal termination 3 per cent)	9
Ectopic pregnancy	6
Miscellaneous obstetric causes	4
Associated causes:	
Cardiac disease	5
Other intercurrent diseases	39
	100

Although most of these headings are clear it may be asked whether unexplained deaths from other causes have not been included under pulmonary embolism. A main heading which does not appear clearly in the table are deaths from anaesthetic difficulties, which contributed in 10 per cent of the headings. The part played by Caesarean section is also hidden — no less than 21 per cent of the deaths followed this operation, performed for a variety of indications.

It has been estimated that in 42 per cent of these deaths there was a factor which was largely avoidable, whether due to the doctor, the midwife, the patient, or to inadequate facilities for antenatal care or care in labour.

Fetal and neonatal mortality
Definitions
A child born before the 28th week is regarded as non-viable and is not included in these statistics (although a few such infants survive).

Stillbirth. Defined as child that does not breathe or show any other sign of life — if the heart is beating the child is not stillborn.

Stillbirth rate: Number of stillbirths per 1000 *total* (live and still) births. Present rate about 10.

Neonatal death rate. Number of infants dying in the first month per 100 *live* births. Present rate about 8.

Infant mortality rate. Number of infants dying during the first year per 1000 *live* births. Present rate about 15.

Perinatal mortality rate. Number of stillbirths and deaths in the first *week* per 1000 *total* births. Present rate under 17.

Causes
As many of the causes of stillbirth may also cause early neonatal death the perinatal mortality is the best index of obstetric care. The cause of a perinatal death can only be properly assessed if both the obstetric history and the autopsy findings are considered. Some causes (e.g., cerebral haemorrhage) may only be proven at autopsy, but on the other hand it is not

helpful to list deaths as due to anoxia (from autopsy findings) unless the cause of anoxia (e.g., antepartum haemorrhage) is given. More than one cause may operate, and if the fetus is macerated histological examination may be impossible. There is not space to list all the causes of perinatal death, and it would be a profitable exercise to compile such a list from preceding pages, but the following factors are especially important:

Low birth weight is not a cause of death, but may contribute to it.

Congenital malformations account for about 19 per cent of perinatal deaths.

Anoxia is the final cause of death in about 15 per cent of perinatal deaths which occur before labour, when it may be due to acute placental lesions such as antepartum haemorrhage, but more gradual placental insufficiency occurs in other cases from pre-eclampsia, diabetes or postmaturity. During labour anoxia, often associated with cerebral trauma, accounts for 26 per cent of perinatal deaths. Such anoxia may be due to compression of the cord, to the placental lesions just mentioned, or may occur during difficult labour from incoordinate uterine action or excessive uterine retraction.

Cerebral haemorrhage is found in 9 per cent of perinatal deaths, often associated with anoxia.

Respiratory distress syndrome (including pulmonary infection) accounts for 12 per cent of first-week deaths.

Infection, either during delivery or afterwards, accounts for some neonatal deaths and contributes to many more.

In addition to these factors the parity, social status and prior nutrition of the mother will have considerable effect on perinatal mortality.

Provision of better facilities, both of staff and equipment, for neonatal paediatric care would reduce the present perinatal mortality and by preventing some forms of handicap would prevent much family unhappiness and social distress, and save a great deal of money.

13

A few historical notes

Caesarean section. *See p. 150.*

Paré, Ambrose, d. 1590. Internal version.

Chamberlen, Peter, d. 1631. Obstetric forceps. *See p. 145.*

Mauriceau, Francois, d. 1709. Jaw and shoulder traction, and much else.

Smellie, William, d. 1763. Mechanism of labour.

Denman, Thomas. Induction of labour, 1756.

Hunter, William, d. 1774. Anatomy of the pregnant uterus.

Rigby, Edward. Accidental and unavoidable haemorrhage, 1775.

Naegele, Franz Karl. Abnormal pelvis, 1839, and much else.

Holmes, Oliver Wendell. Contagiousness of puerperal fever, 1842.

Simpson, Sir James Young. Chloroform, 1847.

Credé, Carl Sigmund Franz. Third stage of labour, 1854, and ophthalmia neonatorum.

Semmelweis, Ignaz Philipp. Puerperal fever, 1861.

Hicks, John Braxton. Uterine contractions of pregnancy, 1872.

Pasteur, Louis. Streptococci and puerperal fever, 1879.

Tait, Lawson. Operation for ectopic pregnancy, 1884.

Hegar, Alfred. Sign of pregnancy, 1895.

Stroganoff, Vasili Vasilievich. Sedative treatment of eclampsia, 1900.

Ballantyne, J. W. Antenatal care, 1901.

Dale, Sir Henry. Pituitary extract, 1909.

Kielland, Christian Caspar Gabriel. Forceps, 1915.

Spalding, Alfred. Sign of fetal death, 1922.

Aschheim, Selmar, and Zondek, Bernard. Biological pregnancy test, 1928.

Moir, Chassar, and Dudley, Harold Ward. Ergometrine, 1935.

Colebrook, Leonard. Prevention of puerperal sepsis, 1936.

Landsteiner, K., and Weiner, A. S. Rhesus factor, 1940.

Malmström, Tage. Perfection of vacuum extractor, 1954.

Donald, Ian. Development of ultrasonic investigation, 1961.

Index

181